Above & Beyond

Above & BEYOND

365 Meditations for Transcending Chronic Pain and Illness

J. S. Dorian

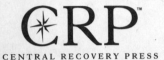

CENTRAL RECOVERY PRESS

CENTRAL RECOVERY PRESS

Central Recovery Press (CRP) is committed to publishing exceptional materials addressing addiction treatment, recovery, and behavioral healthcare topics, including original and quality books, audio/visual communications, and web-based new media. Through a diverse selection of titles, we seek to contribute a broad range of unique resources for professionals, recovering individuals and their families, and the general public.

For more information, visit www.centralrecoverypress.com.

Central Recovery Press, Las Vegas, NV 89129

Publisher: Central Recovery Press
             3321 N Buffalo Drive
             Las Vegas, NV 89129

18 17 16 15 14 13 12   1 2 3 4 5

ISBN-13: 978-1-936290-66-6 (paper)
ISBN-10: 1-936290-66-9

Cover design and interior by Sara Streifel, Think Creative Design

January

January 1

"The only journey is the one within."

RAINER MARIA RILKE

The words *healing* and *curing* are often used interchangeably, although they have separate and distinct meanings. Many of us have had to swallow the bitter reality that for now there is no cure for our condition. However, we can always be healed, through our own efforts or with the help of others.

What do we mean by healing, and how does it differ from curing? In the context of chronic illness, healing relates primarily to one's inner being, to the ways we strive to achieve healthy attitudes as well as personal and spiritual growth. As we progress in these areas, we can gain a positive perspective on our illness, our physical limitations and, indeed, on all of the dramatic changes that have taken place in our lives.

Inner healing can move us from resentment and self-pity to faith and acceptance. The healing process allows us to transcend our fears, to nurture hope, and to face adversity with serenity.

The essence of healing is self-acceptance, through which we affirm our wholeness no matter what our physical condition or how remote the possibility of cure.

THOUGHT FOR TODAY

I will be healed.

"What loneliness is more
lonely than distrust?"

GEORGE ELIOT

Many diseases can be diagnosed rather quickly these days. Certain ones, however, remain elusive and require a considerable amount of detective work. As some of us have discovered, such hard-to-diagnose illnesses can present special problems.

When our symptoms came and went, increased and diminished in severity, and seemed not only mysterious but possibly imaginary, friends, loved ones, and even our physicians became somewhat skeptical. The longer the condition remained undiagnosed and unnamed, the more skeptical some of them became, and the more our own self-doubt grew.

Even now, months after we were finally diagnosed, certain people exhibit a degree of skepticism and mistrust. They raise an eyebrow, so to speak, when we describe our fatigue, pain, and limitations. And then it's as though we are back in pre-diagnosis limbo, frustrated and infuriated.

We'll do everything we can to help those people understand the seriousness of our illness. If it becomes clear that understanding is beyond their reach, we'll then do our best to let it go and move closer to those who do understand.

THOUGHT FOR TODAY

My priorities do not include convincing
skeptics or defending myself.

"We, by our suff'rings,
learn to prize our bliss."

JOHN DRYDEN

As we used to know physical pain, it was something that could always be fixed, not unlike a faulty toaster. We had a rude awakening when *chronic* pain entered our world and threatened to overpower us.

We discovered that doctors can't always determine the cause of pain. Even when technology such as myelograms and CAT scans makes it possible to pinpoint the source and cause of pain, technology can't always relieve pain entirely. So it seemed at first that this lingering pain would wring every bit of joy from our lives.

It has since become clear that there are volumes to learn about pain, and that there is much we can do to understand it, manage it, and limit its influence. One of the most heartening lessons is this: Pain is not simply a physical problem that can be isolated and repaired like a burned-out bulb on a string of Christmas lights. Rather, pain is truly a systems problem involving mind, emotions, attitude, and inner spirit. This means that we need not suffer passively and endlessly; that we can regain control; and that we can marshal our inner resources to achieve transcendence.

THOUGHT FOR TODAY

My goal is not to fix pain but to manage and overcome it.

"Differing but in degree, of kind the same."

JOHN MILTON

Every so often a sense of "uniqueness" comes over me. Recently, for example, in the waiting room of an orthopedic surgeon's office, I felt profoundly different and totally alienated from the other patients who were waiting.

I remember thinking: None of them has the health history and combination of symptoms that I have. Not one of them can possibly understand the kind of life I lead, the problems I have, the difficulties I go through every day.

Not surprisingly, the longer I dwelled on my "uniqueness" the more desperate and disconnected I felt. I had to pull myself back to reality and take the power from those self-destructive thoughts. I did so by looking once more around the waiting room, carefully this time, focusing not on the differences I imagined, but on the similarities.

How can I say that my pain is more severe than anyone else's? How can I insist that my illnesses are more baffling, my symptoms more misunderstood, or my anger and frustration more intense? Why not, instead, concentrate on how much alike we all are, and as the result, benefit from wisdom shared, love exchanged, and hope renewed.

THOUGHT FOR TODAY

Focus on the similarities, not the differences.

"My stronger guilt defeats
my strong intent."
WILLIAM SHAKESPEARE

When I heard the phrase "window of opportunity" in connection with a space-shuttle launch, I could see a clear parallel in my own life. Because of illness, I have a limited amount of energy and often must push through pain in order to get things done. Within each day's window of opportunity I usually choose the activities that provide the biggest payoff and most satisfaction.

Today I chose yoga class over housecleaning. Yesterday I chose gardening over shopping and cooking. The day before yesterday you may have gone to the mall instead of visiting your mother.

The problem is that your enjoyment and satisfaction in the activities you choose are often overshadowed by guilt. You can't help feeling at times that you are being selfish by choosing pleasure over responsibility and self-enrichment over service to others.

But in truth there's no valid reason for you to feel guilty. You're not a selfish person and never have been. This is a very challenging time in your life. Like the space-shuttle astronauts, if you don't take advantage of your windows of opportunity each day, you'll never get off the ground.

THOUGHT FOR TODAY
_____

Doing things for myself is just as important
as getting things done for others.

"Have the courage to face a difficulty,
lest it kick you harder than you bargain for."

KING STANISLAUS OF POLAND

When we get to the point where we fully acknowledge our illness, including its devastating potential, we may think (or wish) that the problems we had before we became sick will fade away. The reality is that preexisting problems may require even *more* of our attention, especially in the area of personal relationships.

For example, if we had constant monetary disagreements with our spouse or partner, the financial strain of illness is likely to increase the burden. Similarly, if we had difficulties communicating, we will probably face even greater communication challenges. The reason is that illness brings up unfamiliar and often frightening feelings for both partners—feelings that need to be expressed and handled.

We may want to take the attitude "I'm too sick to deal with any of this." But we know as adults that we can't abdicate our responsibilities, so we must ignore the temptation to do so. We continue trying to strengthen our relationships, as an integral and valuable part of the healing process.

THOUGHT FOR TODAY

Now, more than ever, we need to work things
out in order to be loving and close.

> "All things are difficult
> before they are easy."
>
> THOMAS FULLER

We've all had the experience of trying to repair something highly fragile or extremely small—replacing the tiny screws in eyeglass frames, for example. As we know, such projects require a steady hand and a delicate touch. Sometimes the harder we try to control our fingers, the more shaky they become; the harder we squint and try to focus, the more our vision blurs.

The same can be true of our inner life. The harder we try to relax, to overcome pain, to achieve inner peace, or to improve our conscious contact with God, the more elusive these objectives become. And all too often, our seeming failure causes us to abandon our efforts in frustration.

However, when we stop trying so hard, when we stop struggling, when we let go and let it happen, we're far more likely to be successful. Rather than "forcing" ourselves to become relaxed, we can unclench our fists and jaws, breathe deeply, and allow the tension to flow out of us. Instead of "battling" our pain, we can calmly return to those control methods that have worked in the past. Instead of straining willfully to move closer to God, we can quietly open ourselves to His loving presence.

THOUGHT FOR TODAY

Let go and let it happen.

"It is easy to live for others; everybody does.
I call on you to live for yourselves."
RALPH WALDO EMERSON

When worsening osteoarthritis in my hips made it necessary for me to start using a cane, my first reaction was a negative one. I saw the cane as a symbol of deterioration rather than a tool that would help me walk more easily and reduce pain. It took me some time to turn my thinking around.

Another obstacle I had to surmount was the reaction of some friends and family members. A few blurted out, "What's the cane for?" or "You're too *young* to use a cane!" Others simply looked at me with an expression of profound sadness. I realized they were upset for two reasons: First, because they didn't want to see me suffering. And second, because a cane didn't fit their image of me as a youthful, active, free-spirited person.

I used the cane for two weeks. Then, responding to other people's reactions and my own self-consciousness, I left it home for two weeks. That hiatus convinced me how necessary and helpful the cane really was. Clearly, I must do what is right for my health, regardless of my own or other people's reactions.

THOUGHT FOR TODAY

I will focus less on self-image and
more on self-healing.

"Better indeed is knowledge than mechanical practice.
Better than knowledge is meditation.
But better still is surrender of attachment to results,
because there follows immediate peace."

BHAGAVAD GITA

After many months, you were finally able to surrender to the painful new realities of your illness. By no means had you been able to achieve total acceptance, yet on a day-to-day basis you had become quite skillful at the fine art of accommodation.

By trial and error, for example, you determined which of your favorite sports you would be able to continue without restriction and which you would have to give up. Similarly, after many enervating swings from one extreme to another, you were able to ration your energy in a balanced way. In short, when you finally understood and accepted your limitations; frustration gave way to the satisfying conviction that you could "live with this illness."

Then, suddenly, a painful and debilitating new symptom pushed you back over the edge into despair. It was as if the rules of the game had been unilaterally and arbitrarily changed; you felt bewildered and betrayed.

Once more, it was necessary to surrender. This time, however, it took days instead of months. And now you've begun to believe, in a most positive way, that life is a series of surrenders through which we achieve transcendence.

THOUGHT FOR TODAY

God never gives me more than I can handle.

"We cannot conquer fate and necessity,
yet we can yield to them in such a manner
as to be greater than if we could."

WALTER SAVAGE LANDOR

On the one hand, we are urged to fight disease with every fiber in our being and with every resource at our command. On the other hand, we are admonished to surrender and seek acceptance. Both approaches make sense, but how can we fight and give up at the same time? The last thing we need these days is another mixed message; we've had all the bewilderments and paradoxes we can handle.

Actually, there is nothing at all contradictory or paradoxical about "fighting" an illness while "surrendering" to it. Fighting an illness isn't like fighting a bear. The object is not to wrestle it to the ground and in the process avoid getting mauled. Rather, the goal in fighting illness is to turn it away or at least stop it in its tracks. "Fighting," in this sense, means garnering our resources, refusing to become a hapless victim, and refusing to give up hope.

"Surrender," in turn, has less to do with giving up than it does with accepting the illness; that is, learning to live fully and gracefully, without self-pity, in the new framework of our life.

THOUGHT FOR TODAY

When I surrender, I do not give up
determination, courage, or hope.
I give up only fear and self-pity.

January 11

> "To question a wise man
> is the beginning of wisdom."
>
> GERMAN PROVERB

Some years ago a biopsy revealed that I had a malignant melanoma. My dermatologist spelled out the deadly nature of this type of cancer and insisted that I undergo surgery immediately.

I was shocked and extremely fearful. My mind raced with speculations and doubts. *Is it really malignant? Could they have mixed up the biopsy results? Is a major excision and plastic surgery really necessary? Will I be cured?*

My family urged me to get a second opinion, but I stalled for several days. Looking back, I now understand my reluctance. Quite frankly, I was afraid that a request for a second opinion would anger my doctor. I didn't want to appear disrespectful, and I certainly didn't want him to think I was questioning his judgment.

The truth, of course, is that good doctors welcome second opinions and are not the least bit threatened by them. If and when they do react poorly, it may be time to consider switching doctors.

By seeking second opinions, we acknowledge that we have choices and can still exercise a certain amount of control over our lives. We begin to take responsibility for our own well-being and become active participants in the treatment and healing process.

THOUGHT FOR TODAY
_____

Whose life is it anyway?

"Experience has taught me this, that we undo ourselves by impatience. Misfortunes have their life and their limits, their sickness and their health."

MICHEL DE MONTAIGNE

For sound and practical reasons, many of us have committed ourselves to living life a day at a time. Experience has taught us that this is the most effective way to remain in the present, and to avoid fearful mental sojourns into the past or future.

However, those among us who suffer from chronic pain can easily become discouraged when applying the one-day-at-a-time approach to rehabilitation, especially if we tend to have more "bad days" than "good days." Because we so desperately want our pain to diminish, we work hard at our healing and rehabilitation programs. We expect to feel better tomorrow or within a few days—certainly by the end of the month—and when we don't, we become disappointed and angry.

The point is that, yes, in many areas we should try to live one day at a time, but in certain illness-related areas it is also important to cultivate a long-term approach. Since the dramatic improvement we seek may not come in eight weeks or eight months, we might be better served by visualizing freedom from pain and its limitations occurring a year, two years, or even three years down the road.

THOUGHT FOR TODAY

High hopes and realistic expectations.

January 13

> "In fair weather prepare for foul."
>
> THOMAS FULLER

Those of us who live in southern California have been told for years that a great earthquake—the big one—could occur at any time, and that we would be well advised to prepare for it. Like many others I ignored the warnings, until the devastating Northridge earthquake literally shook my house off its foundation. Within two weeks I had prepared an elaborate and expensive earthquake survival kit containing all the recommended items and then some.

A year passed. One day, I found myself resenting the time and money I had spent on earthquake supplies that I would almost certainly never use. But then, a short time later, I couldn't help smiling. My negative and rebellious attitude was easy to recognize, for I have felt exactly that same way at times about the effort and money I spend on my health: exercise, stretching, food supplements, medicines, medical tests, and so on.

This time it didn't take an earthquake to shake me back to reality. I realized that while forethought and preparedness rarely bring immediate rewards, they almost always pay off in the long run.

THOUGHT FOR TODAY

Prevention may not always be possible,
but it's always preferable.

"To improve the golden moment of opportunity,
and catch the good that is within our reach,
is the great art of life."
SAMUEL JOHNSON

When we first try a support group, many of us are restrained, skeptical, and cynical. Before we even walk through the door into our first meeting, we take the close-minded view that these people can't possibly help us, because our circumstances are entirely different than theirs.

But then, sometimes within minutes, reluctance gives way to relief; we feel completely at home. As the weeks pass, we benefit in ways we could not have imagined, and our enthusiasm grows.

We soon realize that our case is not different at all, and that we can indeed learn a lot from others with the same illness. How comforting it is to calmly compare and discuss symptoms, options, doctors, and treatments. How freeing it is to dispel myths and acquire new tools for living and coping.

Week after week we are infused with new life as we see others resolving their problems and achieving their goals. Along the way, we receive encouragement and support for our own progress. In no time at all, it seems, our skepticism has given way to loyalty and commitment.

THOUGHT FOR TODAY

There is much I can gain and
much I can give.

January 15

"In the hands of the discoverer, medicine becomes heroic art.... Wherever life is dear he is a demigod."

RALPH WALDO EMERSON

One night in a Chinese restaurant I spotted my cardiologist with his wife and three young children. I caught his eye and waved; he waved back and smiled broadly. Seeing him outside of the usual clinical setting was a comforting reminder of his humanness.

There was a time when I couldn't feel that way. Like most people, I tended to put doctors on pedestals. I ascribed to them far too much power, and for that reason I was afraid of them.

Looking back, I can see how this attitude compromised my medical care. Since I perceived doctors as godlike authority figures, it was important to win their respect and approval. I wanted them to like me and felt they wouldn't if I bothered them by asking too many questions, by calling the office, or by complaining about my symptoms. Only rarely did I question a diagnosis or a recommended course of treatment.

Despite my hard-won enlightenment, those childish feelings occasionally return. When they do, I remind myself that the effectiveness of my medical care depends in large measure on my participation—my objectivity, my honesty, and my assertiveness.

THOUGHT FOR TODAY

Pedestals are obstacles.

"Things are where things are, and, as fate has willed,
So shall they be fulfilled."

AESCHYLUS

When close friends find out about our illness, they often react by saying, "You're such a good person. It's so unfair that this is happening to you!" Our friends and loved ones are insisting, in other words, that it's not right for bad things to happen to good people, and we couldn't agree more.

Such feelings are understandable. If we dwell on them, however, that can make it more difficult for us to accept our illness. If we believe that "good" people shouldn't get sick and die, aren't we implying that it's okay for "bad" people to be afflicted? Aren't we saying, moreover, that illness and death are not natural parts of life but, rather, are eventualities that should befall only those who "deserve" them? And doesn't our "bad things shouldn't happen to good people" philosophy indicate that we see illness and death as punishment?

Unfortunately, we are indeed ill and frequently in pain. Since it is far easier to accept these realities by approaching them as natural parts of life, this might be a good time to examine and perhaps try to change our deep-felt beliefs, attitudes, and feelings on the subject.

THOUGHT FOR TODAY

In God's hands, in God's time.

"Ah, how good it feels!
The hand of an old friend."

HENRY WADSWORTH LONGFELLOW

When it became clear that you would be spending a lot of time in bed, you made the bedroom as comfortable, livable, and as inviting as possible. You bought a firm new mattress and a good reading lamp. You brought in books, plants, and a new TV. You had the windows washed and light-blocking blinds installed.

Now that you're settled into your new environment, you vow that it will be dedicated to wellness rather than illness. Since you don't want to shut yourself off from the world, even though that choice is tempting at times, you decide to put together a support network.

You take out pen and paper and thoughtfully prepare a list. You think first of those people who have already been helpful, who have demonstrated their willingness to be there for you no matter what. Who else? Who among your friends, relatives, and support-group contacts can you truly count on?

Then you make up another list, a shorter one, of the people who can't handle your illness. Finally, you draw up still one more list, not of people, but of the things *you* can do to show your gratitude for the help you are receiving.

THOUGHT FOR TODAY

How can I widen my world?

"It is better to understand little than
to misunderstand a lot."

ANATOLE FRANCE

A friend stopped by to tell my wife and me that she had been diagnosed with a relatively uncommon inflammatory disease. When she mentioned its eight-syllable name, we said we had never heard of it.

"Very few people have heard of it," she responded, "and I get really upset when I try to describe the illness and get them to understand what I've been going through. Some of them look at me blankly. One man at work actually backed away as if he might catch something from me."

Her frustration brought me back to the time, years ago, when I was first diagnosed with Systemic Lupus Erythematosus, commonly known as lupus or SLE. It was all I could do to understand the illness itself, let alone explain it to others. I, too, experienced blank stares and people pulling away.

I eventually came up with a solution to the problem. For some friends and co-workers, I scripted a short explanation that provided just enough information but not more than they needed (or wished) to know. For close friends and relatives, I made copies of an article that explained the illness clearly, concisely, and encouragingly.

THOUGHT FOR TODAY

Explanations aren't always necessary,
but when they are, my guidelines will be
simplicity, clarity, and brevity.

January 19

> "Faith, mighty faith, the promise sees,
> And looks to that alone;
> Laughs at impossibilities,
> And cries it shall be done."
>
> CHARLES WESLEY

Many things were unsettlingly new and different today. We visited a clinic in a strange building in a remote part of town. The nurses and doctors were unfamiliar, and we couldn't help feeling anxious. It again became painfully obvious that cascading and unrelenting change is among the most challenging aspects of chronic illness.

It's not only that we have to deal with new people, new experiences, and new feelings. Many other changes that go far deeper have the potential to traumatize us emotionally, and slow our pace of recovery. We may have to give up a career, seek financial help, and depend on others as never before. We may suddenly have a great deal of time on our hands and face long days and sleepless nights. We may be frightened by the numerous physical changes that are taking place.

But the fear of change diminishes quickly when we affirm the power of God that abides within us. That inner strength allows us to conquer our apprehension and face all changes with courage and confidence. With each new day and each new change, we quietly affirm God's all-knowing, all-powerful, all-loving presence.

THOUGHT FOR TODAY

God will see me through.

"One day, with life and heart,
Is more than time enough to find a world."
JAMES RUSSELL LOWELL

Dawn lightens the sky as it always has. Shadows lengthen and twilight gives way to night in familiar ways. The sun rises and sets with comforting predictability, but the hours in between are another matter entirely. For those of us living with chronic illness, each new day can present unexpected challenges.

We awaken and remain in bed for a while, checking pain levels, wondering how much energy we will have and what we will be able to accomplish. Then fear creeps in and we begin to worry about all sorts of problems. There's a mysterious hum in the refrigerator; a new pothole on the street; a chimney that needs to be cleaned before the weather turns cold.

But we catch ourselves and we push those minor concerns out of our consciousness. The illness has been a teacher; we've begun to recognize what is important and what is not. We have a better sense of what is worthy of our time and what is not.

Today may or may not turn out to be challenging, but it certainly can be special. We resolve not to waste any emotional or physical energy on pettiness and trivialities. We will focus on the important things.

THOUGHT FOR TODAY

How can I best live these new
moments and hours?

January 21

"I am what I am."

ANONYMOUS

Illness often brings with it changes in physical appearance, from temporary skin rashes and hair loss to permanent scarring. Some of the changes are symptoms of the disease; others, including excisions and amputations, are part of the treatment process.

Whether such changes are short-term or permanent, and whether they are relatively minor or profound, they often create a dilemma for us. We can withdraw from social activities because we self-consciously fear other people's perceptions and judgments of us. Or, we can work to bolster our flagging self-image and go on living as normally as possible.

Make-up, wigs, jewelry, hats, and flattering clothing, for example, can go a long way toward improving the way we feel about ourselves. If regular exercise is possible, it also can have a dramatically positive impact on self-image.

But a change in attitude, more than anything, can free us from the pain of self-consciousness and lift us from the depths of despair. Our bodies may have changed—we may be scarred or even skeletal—but we are no less now than we ever were. Indeed, we are more, for each day we face our challenges and transcend them.

THOUGHT FOR TODAY

I may not look the same as before,
but I am no less than before.

> "Nothing is void of God;
> He Himself fills His work."
>
> SENECA

We sometimes refer to the grace of God (often in verbal shorthand: "There but for the grace . . .") when we compare our circumstances with those of others who seem less fortunate. Yet we can tell very little about the reality of God's grace in other people's lives simply by looking at the most obvious aspects of their circumstances—that is, their "outsides."

In truth, God's grace is available to all of His beloved children, not just a "chosen few." We are all equal in His sight; no one among us is more special or deserving than any other. For each and every one of us, God's grace is limitless and ever-present, always available to bring healing power and renewing love.

We often say that God works in mysterious ways. What that means is that His grace can enter and shape our lives in ways that are beyond our comprehension. Isn't it true that many occurrences, which are at first seemingly "bad," often evolve into blessings?

By accepting the grace of God into our lives we can let go of uncertainty and fear. We can accept the good in all situations. We can allow ourselves to be guided toward successful solutions and inner prosperity.

THOUGHT FOR TODAY

I am beloved in His sight.

> "'I can forgive, but I cannot forget,' is only another way of saying, 'I will not forgive.' Forgiveness ought to be like a canceled note — torn in two, and burned up, so that it never can be shown against one."
>
> HENRY WARD BEECHER

It's hard to disagree with the proposition that forgiveness is a powerful force for healing. Many of us know from experience that the act of forgiving can mend relationships, making it possible for love to flow again. Forgiveness can turn the tide of self-destructive negativity and set us free by dissolving toxic and tormenting resentments.

Before we became truly willing to be forgiving, and before we became fully capable of practicing forgiveness, we first had to uncover and discard some of the strange beliefs that were standing in our way. We had long felt, for example, that few acts are sweeter and more satisfying than revenge.

We also had to disavow the notion that proving someone else wrong elevates us in some way. We had to confront and repudiate the belief that some people deserve to be hurt, and that we have a right to manipulate someone with guilt just because he or she wronged us.

Each of these beliefs harmed no one more than ourselves. By accepting this reality and by giving forgiveness the priority it deserves in our lives, we are not only unburdening ourselves but are being healed as well.

THOUGHT FOR TODAY

Perhaps it's time to search out the strange beliefs that are making it difficult for me to forgive myself and others.

"The mind grows sicker than the body
in contemplation of its suffering."

OVID

More than once in recent years I have strongly felt that my body was betraying me. The feeling was of course irrational, but at times I became angry at my surgically repaired heart, at my painfully inflamed joints, and, most frequently, at my immune system for turning against me instead of fighting for me. Needless to say, the longer I held on to the perception that my body was a traitor, the more alienated from myself I became.

When I finally shared these concerns with my close friends in a support group, I received not only empathy but also good advice. I learned that I was self-destructively focusing my anger at my body when I was really angry at the illnesses themselves. As long as my anger was misdirected that way, I couldn't deal with my harmful emotions constructively. As the result of attending the support group, I am now able to clarify and subdue my feelings when such episodes occur.

I've come to an important understanding; that my mind and body are not separate warring entities but rather allies miraculously linked to create the unified whole that is me.

THOUGHT FOR TODAY

Anger at my physical self inhibits rather
than enhances healing.

"It is best to do things systematically,
since we are only human, and
disorder is our worst enemy."

HESIOD

Everything seems to happen at once when there is a medical crisis in the family. It matters little whether we are ill ourselves or we are caregivers—anarchy reigns. We are pulled in many different directions simultaneously, and we are challenged on many levels.

On the physical side there are appointments, treatments, and medications to attend to; there are countless things to do and places to go. We may face powerful new feelings such as despair or terror, as well as uncomfortable old feelings, including guilt and self-pity, which have resurfaced in entirely new ways. At the spiritual level, our faith may be challenged; we may feel let down by God, angry at God, victimized by God.

Clearly, all of this turmoil and pressure must be dealt with, and soon. But how? As simplistic as it may sound, the only way to make progress at each of these levels is to put *first things first*. Instead of diving in impulsively and trying to do everything at once, we must clear our minds, establish priorities, schedule our time, and deal with one thing at a time, one step at a time.

THOUGHT FOR TODAY

Simple solutions are always the best.

"Behold, we know not anything;
I can but trust that good shall fall,
At last — far off — at last, to all
And every winter change to spring."

ALFRED TENNYSON

You were recently diagnosed with a relatively uncommon chronic and progressive disease. Your doctor spelled out the basics and handed you a thick packet of pamphlets and article reprints to help you better understand the illness.

At home, you began reading about debilitating physical and emotional changes that could occur as the disease progresses; the potential effects of the illness on lifestyle, relationships, and sexuality; powerful medications and the possibility of serious side effects. By the time you finished reading a series of bleak case histories, you were in a complete panic.

Later that week, when the shock had worn off, you garnered the courage to reread the material, this time with composure and a degree of acceptance. You then realized that you had focused only on the negative.

You have since been able to absorb all the messages of encouragement: the fact that physical activity helps rather than hurts the condition; the wide array of pain-relieving treatments available; the documented reality that most people with the illness live relatively normal and productive lives; the possibility of spontaneous and complete remission.

THOUGHT FOR TODAY

What about the bright and hopeful side?

> "Mind is the great lever of all things."
>
> DANIEL WEBSTER

When a psychologist friend suggested to me many years ago that there might be a connection between my violent negativity and the tendency of my illnesses to linger, I scoffed. I wondered aloud how he as a medical professional could actually believe something so "blatantly unscientific."

My friend didn't press the point, but he did offer some intriguing examples of the mind's influence over the body. He recounted tales of mentally controlling pain that allowed "firewalkers" to stride across hot coals. He reminded me of a college professor we both had known who died just weeks after the death of his beloved spouse simply because he lost the will to go on living without her.

He talked about a woman who had experienced false pregnancy. There was no growing fetus in her womb, yet she so strongly believed she was pregnant that her mind triggered a wide array of actual physical changes.

Soon after our discussion, I opened myself to the possibility of a mind/body/spirit connection. I've since become a strong believer in that reality, and for years now I have successfully used my own mind and spirit to help in my healing.

THOUGHT FOR TODAY

My most powerful tools for wellness are within.

> "To learn new habits is everything;
> for it is to reach the substance of life."
>
> HENRI FRÉDÉRIC AMIEL

Sometimes it seems that our illness is like a three-ring circus with many acts taking place at once. Of course, we are always in the spotlight. Each day the tyrannical ringmaster, Pain, cracks his whip and forces us to jump through hoops.

We hate being at his mercy, that goes without saying, so over time we've found ways to defer and even defy Pain. Now, instead of having to jump through hoops several times each day, we do so less frequently. It's not a perfect solution, but it's the best we can do right now.

Or is it? Maybe it's time to search for new ways to loosen Pain's hold on us. Maybe it's time to revise our "pain habits" and really break out of our rut.

First, we can open our minds to methods of pain control we haven't yet tried, such as yoga, massage, and creative visualization. Second, we can review our present habits with a medical professional who specializes in pain management. Finally, we can create a new pain management plan by charting the type and degree of pain we experience, the methods we've used for control, and the ones that work best.

THOUGHT FOR TODAY

Pain changes, always. Is the same true
of my responses to it?

"Sleep is better than medicine."

ENGLISH PROVERB

Our ideas about sleep occasionally become convoluted. We begin to think of sleep as a guilty pleasure rather than a vital necessity. We envy men and women who claim to get by on just three or four hours of sleep a night. We then decide that sleep prevents us from fulfilling our daily responsibilities, when in fact just the opposite is true.

In order to overcome such distorted views, we might want to think back to the way we felt after surgery, radiation, or chemo treatments. We were tired all the time, and that wasn't surprising; our wounded bodies needed to be healed and rejuvenated with lots and lots of sleep.

The point is, sleep is not optional. It is a vital healing force that has become more essential than ever in our lives. When we try to "get by" with the same amount of sleep as we did when we were healthy, or try to skimp on sleep because we feel guilty about it, we do ourselves a serious disservice. So let's give ourselves permission, not just once in a while, but every day, to get as much sleep as we need.

THOUGHT FOR TODAY

I will rest, and rest some more, and heal.

"Behavior is a mirror in which
everyone shows his image".

JOHANN WOLFGANG VON GOETHE

Practically every one of us has been upset at one time or another by the insensitive way a close friend or relative is handling our illness. We're surprised that these people aren't more thoughtful and considerate when they're around us, and that they don't try to bend over backwards (just a little) in recognition of what we're going through. But all too frequently they act just the opposite of what we expect. They are often self-centered and display inappropriate or even deplorable behavior.

Wait a minute. Is it realistic to expect that everyone we know will rise to the occasion just because we're seriously ill? Isn't that expecting far too much of them? The true reality is that most people react to serious illness in a manner reflecting their usual style of handling adversity or crisis. Those who tend to be angry respond angrily. Those who see themselves as perennial victims remain victims. Those who are sullen and withdrawn usually stay that way. And those who are usually kind and helpful? Well, they tend to be kind and helpful.

Here again, as in so many areas of life, we are for the most part powerless over other people's attitudes, responses, and behavior. All we can do is state our case clearly and assertively; then let it go and get on with life.

THOUGHT FOR TODAY

Unrealistic expectations cause
unnecessary stress.

January 31

> "Even if it is to be, what end do you serve
> by running to meet distress?"
>
> SENECA

During my first week of recovery from alcoholism I was befriended by a man who had been sober for many years. He urged me to write out a list of my heart's deepest desires, and suggested that I not look at it for at least a year. He said that when I eventually did read the list I would discover that I had greatly short-changed myself; he predicted that the rewards of sobriety would be far greater than anything I could have imagined in those shaky early days. I wish I had drawn up a different kind of list in more recent years; one detailing each fear, worry, and dire projection concerning my various illnesses. That list, too, would be dramatically revealing a year or so down the line.

It would highlight my tendency to torment myself unnecessarily. It would show that most of my fears have nothing to do with the reality of the present and have everything to do with anticipation of the future.

The list would further demonstrate that things rarely turn out as badly as I imagine they will. And it would clearly show that negative thoughts about the future bring unnecessary pain into the present.

THOUGHT FOR TODAY

Fear is the darkroom where all my negatives are developed.

February

February 1

"When one is rising, standing, walking, doing something, stopping, one should constantly concentrate one's mind on the act and the doing of it, not on ones' relation to the act or tis character or value."

ASHVAGOSHA

You have known for a long time that meditation is not only good for the soul but for the physical body as well. Until recently, you followed a comfortable routine, returning day after day to a quiet area where you were able to sit almost motionless for thirty minutes or more at a time, still your mind, and open yourself up to a new awareness. Lately, however, you haven't been able to sit still or remain inactive long enough to meditate in that same way.

You might want to try walking meditation. The very act of walking will allow you to channel your thoughts, providing an array of repetitive motions and sensations on which to focus your mind. There is the measured swing of your arms, the weight shift of your body, the sensations and pressures in your legs as they contact the ground, and, of course, there is the steady rhythm of your breathing.

Then, too, walking will put you in touch with your own life force, always providing something new to see, to hear, to touch, or to smell. Walking, and the meditation that becomes part of it, will sharpen your appreciation of the world around you and inside of you.

THOUGHT FOR TODAY
_____

There are no boundaries or rules for meditation.

"The spirit is the true self, not that physical figure
that can be pointed out by your finger."

CICERO

It has been said that illness redefines us. Indeed, I do get the feeling at times that my illness has taken me over; that I have become the illness and it has become me. It's hard not to actually believe that I am no longer myself.

Even though such feelings are occasionally strong and persistent, it's important for me to remember that they most certainly do not reflect reality. To the contrary, no matter how sick I am, and no matter whether my health improves or declines, I am always myself. My body may change, but my personality, soul, and spiritual core remain as before.

This is not to say that illness hasn't affected my life. It has altered my routines and activities, my relationships, and, of course, the way I feel and think. But deep inside, I am still me.

When I sometimes become demoralized and forget who I am, and what it feels like to be healthy—when I feel that I am again slipping away—I remind myself of an unchanging and comforting reality: In the eyes of my friends and loved ones, and especially in the eyes of God, I remain the same.

THOUGHT FOR TODAY

I am not my illness.

February 3

> "There is so much good in the worst of us,
> And so much bad in the best of us,
> That it hardly behooves any of us,
> To talk about the rest of us."
>
> EDWARD WALLIS HOCH

Every once in a while a pharmaceutical drug is taken off the market because of previously unrecognized (or unacknowledged) toxic side effects. Indeed, at one time or another, many of us have had adverse reactions to even the "safest" of drugs.

Negative attitudes can affect us in the same way. Those of us with chronic illness can be "poisoned" when we indulge in even the smallest of doses.

Few attitudes are more toxic than judgmentalism. We indulge by surreptitiously sniping at other people's decisions, lifestyles, appearances, and the like.

We may feel that we're just "making sport" when we're judgmental in these ways, or that our judgments give us an edge of superiority. But what we're really doing is harming ourselves. This character defect keeps us in a highly stressful state, sending our body's immune system a powerful stream of debilitating messages. Moreover, judgmentalism detours us away from our goals of wellness, spiritual growth, and inner peace.

THOUGHT FOR TODAY

My negative judgments affect *me* negatively.

"We every day and every hour say things of another
that we might more properly say of ourselves."
MICHEL EYQUEM DE MONTAIGNE

It may be difficult to prove scientifically, but many of us know from experience that constant negativity—judgmentalism in particular— weakens our immune system. Moreover, when we unrestrainedly judge others, we tend to feel that we are being judged in the same ways. As a result, we spend a lot of time worrying about what others think of us and we become painfully self-conscious and self-critical. Judgmentalism keeps us angry, afraid, and alienated.

It's easy to say that we'll turn over a new leaf to overcome judgmentalism, but the process takes commitment, effort, and discipline. Over time, we can gradually retrain our minds to notice and appreciate the goodness in others rather than their faults; to focus on the positive instead of the negative; and to be less cynical and more tolerant.

We can also acknowledge that the flaws we see and criticize in others are probably the same traits that we dislike in ourselves. At the same time we can concentrate on our spiritual goals, reminding ourselves regularly that God loves each and every one of us unconditionally. And we can strive to live in that same spirit, as we believe He would have us live.

THOUGHT FOR TODAY

Judgmentalism leaves no room
for healing and growth.

February 5

> "Know thyself."
>
> INSCRIPTION ON THE TEMPLE TO APOLLO AT DELPHI

Many spiritual philosophies describe a special part of a person called the "observer." It's the part of us that can witness feelings and thoughts as they surface, pass through our minds, and float away—without reacting to them.

In recent years, I have been able to use meditative practice to come to terms with my various illnesses and, at times, transcend them. When I am able to separate myself from negative thoughts and emotions such as fear and resentment, and from uncomfortable physical experiences such as pain and fatigue, I affirm once again that I am much more than my body, my illness, or my thoughts.

Looking at it another way, chronic illness has given me the opportunity to enlarge my identity. I have gradually been able to discover and explore new dimensions of myself—my inner spirit, my essence, my soul, and the presence and power of God within.

Those who suffer from chronic illness wonder from time-to-time if there is a meaning or purpose for their suffering and, of course, each of us must find our own answers to this question. I have come to believe that illness is a spiritual teacher. As a result of these teachings my life has taken on new meaning.

THOUGHT FOR TODAY

I am so much more than my illness.

> "Feed your faith, and doubt
> will starve to death."
>
> ANONYMOUS

In the early stages of illness, we vowed that we would do everything possible to halt the progress of our disease and heal. Spirituality was high on our list of priorities. We believed that a Higher Power could help us get well and we felt that prayer and meditation would bring us closer to that goal.

Along the way, some of us were sidetracked by the unspoken yet persistent thought that God was somehow responsible for our illness. Maybe He was punishing us, or perhaps He simply didn't care. Either way, we felt that at times God had let us down—and we were angry at Him.

Not surprisingly, these confused feelings weakened our trust, and prevented us from fully availing ourselves of God's power and love. During that trying period, it was difficult to put our faith to work.

When we finally shared these feelings with close friends or spiritual advisors, we were gently reminded that the dilemma was of our own making. The reality of God hadn't changed; nor had His divine plan for our ultimate well-being. His unconditional love for us was as strong as ever. The only thing that had *temporarily* changed, influenced by illness, was our perception of God.

THOUGHT FOR TODAY

Forever and ever, God is on
my side and at my side.

February 7

> ## "Modest doubt is called
> ## the beacon of the wise."
> WILLIAM SHAKESPEARE

Now that we're sick, we have to learn to care for ourselves in entirely new ways. Often, we wonder if we're "doing it right." We fret about mistakes we may have made, and we agonize about tasks we are no longer able to undertake or promises we are unable to keep.

We berate ourselves for occasionally giving in to our cravings for certain foods, knowing they are the worst possible things we could eat. We feel guilty when we allow ourselves to sleep all day. But we hate to wake up, because at least when we're asleep we're not in pain. We torment ourselves when we're not in the best mood or when we haven't been able to control our disposition.

When we have these painful feelings, let's try to remember that there is no "correct" way to experience illness. If there is a common denominator in every illness, it is *uncertainty*. Nevertheless, we can always reach out for advice, strive to achieve balance in every area, and do our very best each day to maintain self-respect and dignity.

THOUGHT FOR TODAY

Am I adding to my burdens
by doubting myself?

"They must often change who would be
constant in happiness or wisdom."

CONFUCIUS

Some of us occasionally excuse our childish or inappropriate behavior by thinking or saying, "Well, that's just the way I am. I can't help it." When illness has us in its thrall, we may be tempted to fall back on that self-serving rationalization more frequently.

When pain and fatigue are especially acute, we probably should relax normal restraints to some extent. However, that doesn't mean we should allow ourselves unlimited behavioral latitude when we're feeling poorly.

By thinking or saying, "That's just the way I am, I can't help it," aren't we really telling ourselves that we can't change and won't ever change? Aren't we insisting that we have no choice or power concerning our emotions and behavior? And, in order to justify self-will running riot, aren't we making it clear that we're quite willing to accept these self-imposed limitations?

No matter how severe or debilitating a physical illness may be, we always have some control over our attitudes and actions. We *always* have choices. And we *always* have spiritual tools which, when applied, allow us to meet life with an unbound and tranquil spirit.

THOUGHT FOR TODAY

I can change, but first I have
to be willing to change.

February 9

> "The man with insight enough to admit his limitations comes nearest to perfection."
>
> JOHANN WOLFGANG VON GOETHE

Your mom called today to confirm plans for dinner and a movie tomorrow night. Your initial response was, "Great, I'm looking forward to it." But then common sense overrode your enthusiasm. You realized you couldn't predict how you would be feeling tomorrow, so you told your mother you'd have to let her know in the morning.

Later, you began to feel sad and demoralized. You hated to make your mother wonder and worry. You hated having to leave the plans up in the air. And those feelings were intensified because you've always taken pride in your ability to keep commitments, and because you've always felt good about being dependable and responsible.

Times are changing, and clearly so. And from now on you are going to do your best, as gracefully as possible, to change along with them. You'll try to be as understanding and as patient with yourself as others have been with you. You'll fight off the idea that you have suddenly become irresponsible, undependable, or unstable. You'll remind yourself that today's limitations have nothing at all to do with the kind of person you are.

THOUGHT FOR TODAY

The illness affects my body,
not my values or moral fiber.

> "He prepares to go mad with
> fixed rule and method."
>
> HORACE

It was 2:00 a.m., and the sound of the electric drill awakened my wife. When she came into the living room I explained that I was bolting the bookcase to the wall to prevent it from falling during the next earthquake. "It's been on my list for a long time," I added feebly. She shook her head with dismay and suggested I finish in the morning.

The incident forced me to take a hard look at my willingness to be tyrannized by "to do" lists. It occurred to me that each notation on my list usually begins as a random thought. By writing it down and prioritizing it, I transform the simple thought into an urgent necessity. I realized then why I so often feel driven, anxious, and frustrated without knowing why.

Since "The Night of the Bookcase," as my wife and I have come to call it, I've been trying to change my ways. First, I endeavor to view my thoughts as thoughts and *nothing more*. Second, I try to step back from the thought, so to speak, in order to objectively weigh its importance. After that, I'm ready to decide whether the thought is worth acting on.

THOUGHT FOR TODAY

Are my daily "to do" lists putting
me under needless pressure?

> "The foundations which we would dig
> about and find are within us, like the
> Kingdom of Heaven, rather than without."
>
> SAMUEL BUTLER

In each of our lives there is at least one very special person. There is that marvelous doctor, never at a loss for a wise and reassuring response to our concerns. There is that nurse who is so empathetic and encouraging. There is the therapist who listens patiently and helps us sort out and deal with our emotions. There is the spouse or partner who is loving and supportive beyond the call of duty.

It's easy to become attached to and dependent on certain individuals who care for us when we are ill and in pain. As we well know, however, few things are permanent, including treasured relationships. Doctors are transferred or retire. Nurses change shifts. Partners sometimes move on. When such separation occurs, it's understandable for us to feel lost, alone, or even forsaken.

At such times we can turn within and find the very same qualities we had looked for and depended on in others. We can turn to God, our ultimate and unwavering source of love, comfort, and strength. In sickness and in health, for better or for worse, forever and ever, we can depend on God.

THOUGHT FOR TODAY

I can count on God.

> "Insensible of mortality and desperately mortal."
>
> WILLIAM SHAKESPEARE

I try not to pay much attention to survival statistics for people with life-threatening illnesses. Yet the numbers do reflect some sort of reality, and they're hard to ignore entirely. The longevity tables for survivors of cardiac bypass surgery and malignant melanoma, in particular, have forced me to come to terms with my own mortality. And this awakening has brought me closer to God in a way I never thought possible.

It's not that I lacked faith before those illnesses struck. I began developing a relationship with God in the first years of my recovery from alcoholism, and for more than two decades now I have tried to draw closer to Him.

But coming face to face with the actual possibility of death has deepened my faith, allowing me to have a truly trusting relationship with God, the kind I had long sought but somehow couldn't quite achieve.

The truth is, I have no idea how long I'm going to live. It could be three more years or twenty more years. My doctors and I will do all we can to keep me around for a long time, but ultimately it's in God's hands. And that is a deeply comforting reality.

THOUGHT FOR TODAY

God has a plan for my life
and its foundation is love.

"Give us grace to listen well."

JOHN KEBLE

We run into an old friend whom we haven't seen for months. He is pale and seems far thinner than we remember. After we exchange pleasantries, he confides that he has been quite ill and is suffering with chronic pain.

Even as he speaks and tries to hold our gaze, we can feel our attention wavering. Questions, ideas, and potential advice for him crystallize quickly in our mind: *How did they diagnose it? Did you get a second opinion? Anti-inflammatory medications don't work for that. The things that helped me were meditation and yoga. I should lend him that book I like so much and put him in touch with my pain specialist.*

We're tempted to interrupt his description of the illness and its effects so that we can pass along our words of wisdom. But we stop ourselves. We remember what it felt like to be interrupted when we were telling someone about our illness. We remember what it felt like to be besieged with advice and admonitions, to be coaxed to do this and cautioned not to do that. All we really wanted was someone to listen to us, just to listen and let us talk.

THOUGHT FOR TODAY

If there's no listening, there's no compassion.

"Patience and diligence, like faith,
remove mountains."

WILLIAM PENN

Patience has never been one of our strong points, although we've certainly advanced far beyond the "gimme, gimme, right now!" hysterics of childhood. It's a lot easier to wait our turn, to tolerate other people's mistakes, and, in general, to remain calm when circumstances or the actions of others fail to meet our expectations or timetables.

But when it comes to our illnesses, we all too often revert back to childlike impatience. A new medication is prescribed, for example, and if we don't feel significantly better right away, we become discouraged. When our pain hasn't diminished after a few sessions of physical therapy, we're ready to throw in the towel. If we don't see immediate benefits from meditation, we give it up.

If we've had chronic pain for months or years, it's hardly reasonable to expect it to disappear in just a few days just because we're taking a new drug or practicing a new therapy. When we do grow quickly discouraged let's remember that the road to wellness and recovery is sometimes a long one, and not always a straight one. If we remain committed, consistent, faith-filled—and *patient*—our hard work will more likely pay off.

THOUGHT FOR TODAY

It's worth the effort—and the wait.

> "As the inner vision is awakened, one comes to know one's own home, deep within the self."
>
> SRI GURU GRANTH SAHIB

During a visit to Rome years ago, I had the opportunity to view Michelangelo's stunningly lifelike and luminescent sculpture, *La Pieta*. Later, when I tried to describe the masterpiece to an artist friend, he told me that Michelangelo had a detailed inner vision of the completed work long before he first took hammer and chisel to the huge block of marble.

We, too, can rely on inner visions to help us build our lives, especially at those times when we temporarily veer off the path of healing and become disillusioned and confused. We need not be artists or even think of ourselves as creative individuals in order to develop inner visions and then bring them to reality.

An inner vision of capability can eventually lead to self-assurance, confident decision-making, and the ability to again see ourselves right-sized.

An inner vision of wellness can begin to manifest itself in greater acceptance, positive attitudes, and renewed hope.

An inner vision of harmony can bring an end to conflict and discord and mark the beginning of peace of mind.

THOUGHT FOR TODAY

The best of me is within.

"Seize the day!"

HORACE

As soon as you opened your eyes this morning, you knew that extreme pain would be your constant companion all day. You lingered in bed, allowing your mind to fully awaken along with your body, getting in touch with past experiences of days such as this. You recalled episodes of pain-generated impatience and fury. You remembered, all too clearly, how your negativity and irritability manifested itself in behavior so hurtful that it sometimes brought others to tears.

So you remained in bed a while longer, taking the time to decide that this would not be that kind of day. You vowed to be as accepting as possible of your pain without the pressure of unrealistic expectations. You reminded yourself that your loved ones are hurting right along with you, and that they need your patience and compassion just as much as you need theirs.

You affirmed the realities that pain diminishes and eventually passes, that help is always close at hand, and that you need not suffer silently or sullenly. You promised yourself that you would reach out to fellow sufferers and to God.

THOUGHT FOR TODAY

Pain or no pain, how do I choose
to live this day?

"We can only learn to know ourselves and do what we can—namely, surrender our will and fulfill God's will in us."

ST. TERESA OF AVILA

It is critically important for us to fight the disease with all of our strength and resources. However, in the broader realm of our life it is just as essential to *stop* fighting everyone and everything else.

How can we achieve this state of surrender that leads to inner tranquility? One of the best ways is to consciously and conscientiously seek and do God's will rather than heedlessly or bullishly following the dictates of our own will.

There are various pathways to spiritual surrender including prayer, meditation, structured solitude, and working with a spiritual advisor. Some people feel that God's will is often expressed through intuition. Intuition is your "inner voice," which exists independently of intellect and ego.

How can we be certain, day by day, that our will is in alignment with God's will? More than likely we will be able to tell, over time, by a powerful sense that we are "going with the flow." If most of the time we feel tranquil and in harmony with others and the world around us, these are good indications that we are following God's will. But if we are frequently in conflict—if we feel anxious, irritable, and fearful—these are good indicators that we are being motivated primarily by self-will.

THOUGHT FOR TODAY

Spiritual surrender leads to serenity.

"May you live all the days of your life."

JONATHAN SWIFT

When the illness made its presence known, it was unwelcome, clearly so, yet it rudely shouldered its way into every corner of our lives. We were told that the course of the disease would be determined by our response to surgery, to drug therapy, to radiation, and that an equally important factor would be our *attitude*.

Whether we are seriously ill ourselves or caring for someone with cancer, AIDS, or Alzheimer's, if we haven't done so yet, we will have to make a highly critical choice. If we see the illness as a death sentence, then our choice is to position ourselves at death's door, waiting fearfully and despondently for the end. With this choice we give up the opportunity to grow closer than ever with loved ones. We also forgo the process of living in the precious time remaining in our lives.

If, however, we choose to regard the illness as one of life's most challenging chapters, rather than a death sentence, our experience and involvement can be productive and fulfilling. By embracing and treasuring the time we have together, searching for meaning and significance in each new day, we transcend illness and actively cherish the gift of life.

THOUGHT FOR TODAY

Would I rather spend my time fearing
death or embracing life?

February 19

I know that I'm not supposed to keep prescription drugs after their expiration dates. But like so many people I often neglect to throw them away, even though they are no longer effective or even appropriate for my illnesses. When I decided to get rid of a drawer full of outdated medications not long ago, I found myself lingering morosely over their names, dosages, and the month and year they were prescribed.

Before I flushed them away I tried, with little success, to remember which drugs had been prescribed for what conditions. What I did remember vividly were the terrible side effects of some—the nausea, vertigo, headaches, and rashes; the outlandish $3-a-pill cost of several; the complete ineffectiveness of so many. And I thought despairingly, "What a waste! No more drugs, no more pills, never again. The hell with it."

That evening, when I became willing to let go of my self-destructive anger, I was restored to sanity. I recommitted myself, deep in my heart, to continue doing whatever I can and whatever it takes to get well again.

THOUGHT FOR TODAY

Medicines are not panaceas but tools
to help me build my house of health.

"For life, with all it yields of joy and woe . . . Is just
a chance o' the prize of learning love."
ROBERT BROWNING

A young friend burst into tears as she described a cross-country visit to her dying father. She had rushed to his side as the family "savior," expecting to take charge of his medical care, bring him comfort, and unify her grieving family. "My dad was glad to see me," she said, "but he made it emphatically clear to everyone that he wanted to be left alone. I'm shattered."

We each choose to deal with critical or terminal illness in our own way. Some of us require a great deal of family involvement while others want very little attention. However, these highly personal choices are not always easy to make, since every person in the family circle has special emotional needs during times of crisis.

Those of us who are ill must nevertheless set our own priorities. If we need to be alone, even though our loved ones insist on being constantly at our side, we should stick to our guns.

We understand how difficult it can be for family members to comply with our wishes to be left alone. If possible, we can explain the way we feel and try to help them respect our needs and wishes.

THOUGHT FOR TODAY

Right now, in spite of emotional pressures from loved ones, I need to do what's right for me.

February 21

> "The future is purchased by the present."
>
> SAMUEL JOHNSON

"We're going to get this thing under control," the doctor assures you. For the first time in months you're able to smile through the pain. She then outlines a rigorous program designed to relieve your crippling joint inflammation and stiffness.

For two weeks after that you follow the program religiously. You set your watch alarm in order to take each of the four medications on time, and you carefully weigh out the diet supplements. You take frequent rest periods, stretch and exercise as prescribed, and do your utmost to eliminate stress from your life. Then, one exhausting day, with no real improvement evident or in sight, you are suddenly overwhelmed with the prospect of continuing this demanding routine for the rest of your life.

Join the club. Many of us experience disillusionment when we optimistically plunge ahead with a new treatment regimen and then discover how difficult and time-consuming it is.

But there are many ways to reverse such self-doubt and waning motivation. Perhaps the very best way is to take a hard look at the consequences of giving up the treatment program, or doing it haphazardly, and allowing the disease to resume its debilitating course.

THOUGHT FOR TODAY

Haven't you felt bad enough, long enough?

"Let the soul be joyful in the present,
disdaining anxiety for the future, and tempering
bitter things with a serene smile."

HORACE

It takes more than fear of getting sicker to remain committed to a rigorous treatment program. It also takes more than guts and willpower to get us through. However, assuming that recovery is our overriding priority, there are a number of other approaches and actions that can help us achieve our goal of commitment.

First, and foremost, let's put aside the panic-producing idea that we have to follow the program "for the rest of our lives." We need only concern ourselves with today, remembering that we can remain committed to almost anything one day at a time.

It helps a lot to establish a daily routine. At the same time, we should allow ourselves a certain amount of flexibility, considering not only the fact that we are human, but also that illness sometimes takes unexpected turns. Another way to ease the pressure of a time-consuming regimen is to combine certain activities: exercise and meditation, for example, or stretching and TV-watching.

If we follow these and other confidence-building approaches, before long we will find that we look forward to our daily routine and to the rewards of certain activities in particular.

THOUGHT FOR TODAY

My treatment program isn't a
punishment, but a promise.

February 23

> "Lord, grant that I might not so much
> seek to be loved as to love."
>
> ST. FRANCIS OF ASSISI

Through our struggles against illness we've learned more about love than in all the previous years of our lives. In the past, many of us took love for granted. We gave and received love but rarely thought about its effects on others and ourselves. As an action and emotion, love was pleasurable and desirable, and that was pretty much the extent of it.

Recently we have discovered the incredible healing power of love. We have become convinced, in fact, that nothing in a person's wellness program is more important than love. We have found that the more love we have in our lives, the more quickly we tend to heal, the more likely we are to remain well, and the better we feel.

Love is not just a potent force for physical healing but for emotional and spiritual healing as well. When illness brings on feelings of unworthiness, for example, or distances us from God, the love we receive and accept from others—and the love we give to them—helps us overcome those feelings as if by magic.

THOUGHT FOR TODAY

My new prescription, with unlimited refills,
will be boundless love.

> "Even now I am full of hope,
> but the end lies in God."
>
> PINDAR

Not long ago, when my illnesses seemed to be feeding on each other and I was in constant pain, I became quite depressed. Fearful thoughts began to take root: My cancer is in remission right now, but will it stay that way? My lupus has been getting progressively worse, so what's it going to be like next year or five years from now? And what about the bypass grafts in my coronary arteries? Will they remain clear?

Those uncertainties plagued me for days. It soon occurred to me that my loved ones could well be tormented by the same unanswerable questions.

And that was exactly the point, I realized one bright morning; those kinds of questions *are* unanswerable. In order to rise above my depression, I would have to rekindle the hope that had sustained me in the past. I began by contacting friends who had survived the same illnesses. They reminded me that technology moves steadily forward, ever closer to new treatments and cures.

But ultimately it became a very personal matter between God and me. It became, and remains, a reaffirmation of my faith that He will care for me and watch over me *always*.

THOUGHT FOR TODAY

In all the uncertainty, there is
one Great Certainty.

February 25

> "Loneliness breaks the spirit."
>
> JEWISH PROVERB

Many a sad song has been sung about loneliness. Indeed, probably as many poems, plays, paintings, and novels have been inspired by loneliness as by love; there is nothing as heart-wrenching as feeling all alone, even in a crowd.

While loneliness may inspire creativity, those of us with chronic illness who regularly experience the feeling find nothing inspiring or even interesting about its advent. To the contrary, loneliness almost always brings with it self-pity, depression, and despair.

However, many of us are finding that we no longer have to feel alone, no matter what our circumstances. All it takes to restore a sense of connectedness is the willingness to reach out, especially to others who are similarly challenged.

We are doing so in very practical ways, using telephone help-lines and attending support group meetings. We are also reaching out with our minds and hearts, reflecting on the reality that at this very moment, in places all over the world, there are other people in exactly the same situation with the very same feelings. We are not alone and need not feel alone ever again.

THOUGHT FOR TODAY

I am not alone.

> "Let not your mind run on what you lack
> as much as on what you have already."
>
> MARCUS AURELIUS

When I was nine years old I decided to run away from home. Although I had no particular destination in mind, I spent several hours filling a cigar box with things I thought necessary for my survival, including a Boy Scout knife, matches, safety pins and rubber bands, bubble gum, some coins, and a pair of shoelaces.

It hadn't occurred to me to bring food, so I didn't get very far. Perhaps that's why, when I started traveling as an adult, I invariably prepared a lengthy packing list. My suitcases bulged not only with necessities, but also with items for every imaginable contingency.

Over the years I've gradually been able to lighten my burden. I've learned that the most important thing I need, in any and all situations, can always be found deep within me. That is where I can find reassurance, courage, strength, and peace. That is where I can always find God.

No matter where I go or what I do, and no matter what is occurring in my life, His limitless grace is always available. Whenever I choose, whenever I am willing, I focus on that inner reservoir. I breathe deeply and let the peace rise.

THOUGHT FOR TODAY

I have everything I need.

February 27

"Look up, laugh loud, talk big, keep the color
in your cheek and the fire in your eye,
adorn your person, maintain your health,
your beauty, and your animal spirits."

WILLIAM HAZLITT

How long has it been since something struck you so funny that you laughed until your ribs ached and your eyes watered? Has it been far too long? Does it seem that nothing is even slightly amusing anymore?

Perhaps, because you feel so fragile, you work hard to hold your emotions in check and are unwilling to become too sad or too glad. Perhaps, because of lingering illness, you frequently feel blue and it seems there is no place for humor in your life. Or perhaps, because of the way your loved ones are being affected by your illness, you think that laughter would be inappropriate.

For now, let's put all of that aside. Let's forget about maintaining our composure and keeping a stiff upper lip. Let's remember how wonderful it feels to release ourselves in uproarious laughter, to giggle, snort, and even bellow at the absurdity of our own foibles, malapropisms, and indelicacies. Let's remember, above all, that few healing forces are more accessible or powerful than the sound and sensation of our own laughter.

THOUGHT FOR TODAY

I'm laughing not just to keep from crying
but also for pleasure and peace of mind.

"When a resolute young fellow steps up to
the great bully, the world, and takes him boldly
by the beard, he is often surprised to find it
comes off in his hand, and that it was only tied
on to scare away the timid adventurers."

RALPH WALDO EMERSON

We've all been people-pleasers at one time or another in our lives. Some of us still have trouble standing up for ourselves. We fear disapproval from others; we don't want to be out of step or look bad. In short, we've never learned to say no and then stick by our guns.

In the past, the consequences were not always negative when we caved in to pressure from others. Now that we're ill, however, we simply can't afford to participate in activities that may not be in our best interest. So we're putting our people-pleasing days behind us. We're learning to say "no," gracefully, but firmly.

We're aware that some people automatically take a no response as rejection and become hurt. That's why, whenever possible, we're honest about our reason for turning down an invitation or bowing out of a commitment. If it seems appropriate, we express our appreciation for the offer.

Of course, it's almost impossible to be appreciative (or even graceful) when someone puts on the pressure. On those occasions, it is especially important to stand our ground. The more often we're able to say no and experience positive results, the easier it gets.

THOUGHT FOR TODAY

Do I still hesitate to say no for fear of disapproval?

March

"Wonder and amazement inhabits here."

WILLIAM SHAKESPEARE

When I once asked a urologist to prescribe something for a minor bladder infection, he said he'd prefer to wait a few days. By way of explanation, he asked me if I knew where the world's best pharmacy was located. When I shrugged, he smiled and said, "Inside your own body."

The doctor used the immune system as one example, extolling its miraculous ability to regulate the body and fight off infection and disease.

On days when a lupus flare-up causes my own immune system to attack the body it is supposed to defend, I think back to that conversation about my "inner pharmacy." I do so in order to transcend the pain and keep hope alive.

I remember times in childhood when I'd be out running and playing just one day after a high fever had kept me in bed. I remember my recovery from an auto accident, and how well my bones knit and my wounds healed. I recall adrenaline rushes that saved my life; the reassuring sight of blood quickly coagulating; the endorphin rewards following exercise. I reflect on *all* of my body's incredible capabilities and, as ever, I am awed and grateful.

THOUGHT FOR TODAY

The miracle of self-healing is occurring at this very moment.

March 2

> "I, who have never willfully pained another,
> have no business to pain myself."
>
> MARCUS AURELIUS

It seems that we are being tested these days. We may know intellectually that this is not the case, but we can't help feeling that our ability to cope and endure is constantly being examined and gauged.

We wonder (and we sense that people around us are wondering, too) just how much longer we'll be able to get by with night after night of pain-interrupted sleep. We worry that we won't make the grade in adjusting to new limitations and rapidly changing relationships. We fear that we won't be able to push through pain or even remain hopeful in the days and weeks ahead.

Let's pull back! Let's take a break from the demanding "pass-fail" mindset we've created for ourselves. Let's put aside all of that punishing self-criticism and self-judgment. Let's free our minds of wonder, worry, and fear.

Instead, let's fill our minds and hearts with total acceptance of God's grace. God's love for us is not contingent on how we "measure up" or whether or not we "make the grade." God's love for us is eternal and unconditional.

THOUGHT FOR TODAY

My recovery and wellness programs
are not pass-fail propositions.

"Seeing that a Pilot steers the ship in which we sail, who will never allow us to perish even in the midst of shipwrecks, there is no reason why our minds should be overwhelmed with fear and overcome with weariness."

JOHN CALVIN

I know that when I harbor negative thoughts in my mind long enough, repeating them over and over and letting them roll around in my consciousness, the thoughts become distressing feelings. And when I dwell on those feelings, allowing them to mushroom within me, they often manifest themselves in hurtful words and actions toward myself or others.

My goal today is to prevent negative thoughts from influencing the way I see myself and the way I live my life. While it will be impossible to eliminate such thoughts entirely, I can deliberately choose to reverse them, transform them, or seek their opposite when they do surface.

Instead of dwelling on physical, mental, or circumstantial limitations, I will focus on God's larger world and all it has to offer.

Instead of criticizing the things that are wrong or lacking among my friends, family members, and healthcare team, I will acknowledge and appreciate their concern, love, and fundamental desire for my well-being.

Instead of allowing fear to take root and grow wild within me, I will open myself to the protecting presence of God, going forward again with courage and confidence.

THOUGHT FOR TODAY

I will not give power to negative thoughts.

March 4

> "It is wonderful how quickly you get used
> to things, even the most astonishing."
>
> EDITH NESBITT

It used to be that we did pretty much what we wanted, when we wanted. Apart from family and financial responsibilities, we were able to "rip and run" as we pleased and to schedule our activities by whim.

Those days may not be gone forever, but unfortunately we haven't experienced them in a while. Chronic illness has reined us in sharply, and on some days pain hobbles us to the point of immobility.

What we've learned to do, in response to chronic illness, is to listen carefully to our bodies' signals and messages. Through meditation, body scans, stretching exercises, yoga, and similar techniques, we "check in, tune in, and listen in" and then act on what we learn.

As a primary example, we're becoming increasingly familiar with our daily body rhythms. We're discovering when our energy levels are generally highest and lowest, and how to plan activities accordingly.

In my own case, I now know that my best hours are from mid-morning to mid-afternoon. Then I can expect a letdown, followed by a surge after dinner. So I've learned to make the most of the high-energy times, and to accept and respect the low-energy ones.

THOUGHT FOR TODAY

When I seek and follow my body's
guidance, then I am at my best.

> "Let other pens dwell
> on guilt and misery."
>
> JANE AUSTEN

Those close to us can't help knowing what we've been going through; it would be impossible for us to hide the effects of the disease. Sometimes, however, we try to smile through the pain, hoping they'll think we're doing fine. At other times we shut ourselves away in order to spare our loved ones the anguish they so obviously feel.

Most of the time, though, we're honest and open about our symptoms because we know how important it is for all of us to be as accepting as possible. The problem is that we frequently feel terribly guilty for causing our family members so much heartache.

We feel guilty? Why guilt, of all things? It isn't as if we brought the illness on ourselves. It isn't as if we can "will" ourselves back to health. It isn't as if we're responsible for the ways our loved ones react to the illness, or that we have any control over their reactions.

The point is that there are quite enough weighty issues in our life these days, and most of them are as unavoidable as they are unfathomable. Guilt, however, is another story entirely. It is one burden we *don't* need to pick up and carry around.

THOUGHT FOR TODAY

Guilt is bad medicine.

March 6

> "Aging seems to be the only
> available way to live a long life."
>
> DANIEL FRANÇOIS ESPRIT AUBER

"It's tough getting old, isn't it?" That's what we hear, all too often, when we get into a conversation with someone about our illness. Whether we are twenty-seven or seventy-two, we usually respond by smiling and agreeing. And for the moment that seems to take the focus off us and put the matter to rest.

For most of us, there is little purpose in challenging such a remark. Whether such a remark is tossed out blithely (as it usually is) or taken seriously, what really matters is our own beliefs about illness and age.

Although some illnesses are age-related, many are not. In my case, I see illness and age as entirely separate issues, and I refuse to let illness "make me" act, think, or feel old.

Moreover, I'm not about to start "acting my age" just because I'm ill, nor will I allow my age to set me apart from others, younger or older. Illness notwithstanding, I believe that age has more to do with attitude and inner spirit than numbers, actuarial or otherwise. In short, I'm as young or as old as I choose to be.

THOUGHT FOR TODAY

The substance and quality of my life have
very little to do with the year of my birth.

> "Fear makes men ready
> to believe the worst."
>
> QUINTUS CURTIUS RUFUS

You'll be going back to work in a couple of weeks, and you're more nervous than on that day five years ago when you were first hired. You are not afraid that you can't do the work; it's not that. Nor are you afraid, as you were back then, that your performance won't match the promises on your resume.

What does concern you is how your co-workers will react to your illness and behave toward you. Will they treat you as before? Or have some of them fallen prey to such myths as: Cancer makes workers less efficient. Cancer is contagious. Cancer is a death sentence.

Here again, as with so many aspects of illness, careful planning and clear communication can smooth the way, solve any actual problems, and forestall potential new ones.

If you haven't kept up contact during your treatment and recovery—a few phone calls will ease your co-workers' concerns about you and give you the chance to dispel any misconceptions they may have— once you're back at work, you may want to schedule a get-together with fellow employees. This get-together will allow them (and you) to air concerns, correct wrong ideas, and decide the best ways to work together again.

THOUGHT FOR TODAY

I will ground my thoughts in reality, imagining the best rather than the worst.

"Knowledge is of two kinds: we know a subject ourselves
or we know where we can find information upon it."

SAMUEL JOHNSON

I decided, not long ago, that it was time to rearrange my bookshelves. I made excellent progress until I reached the shelf reserved for books, pamphlets, and materials pertaining to my various illnesses, namely heart disease, cancer, lupus, alcoholism, and osteoarthritis.

As I looked through the material, I was immediately struck by the rapid pace of change in diagnostic criteria, treatment approaches, and technology. The newspaper clippings, in particular, showed me how quickly a so-called medical breakthrough can be set aside or repudiated.

Browsing further, it became clear to me that at least half the material I had gathered was already obsolete. Probably an additional 25 percent was well on the way to becoming outdated.

The experience drove home once again the importance of self-education and the need to continually search out the very latest medical information, while avoiding literature that is several years behind the times, misleading, and possibly even dangerous. I now rely less on my own haphazardly gathered medical source materials and more on information available through support organizations, university bookstores, government agencies, and on-line computer services.

THOUGHT FOR TODAY
_____
Staying up to date is my responsibility.

"God! Thou art love!
I build my faith on that."

ROBERT BROWNING

When illness comes to visit it often brings with it a considerable amount of baggage. One suitcase may overflow with an emotion-packed "Why me?" Another may be crammed with messages like, "I deserve to be sick!" Still another may be packed solid with, "I'm half the person I used to be" notions.

There are those who try to get rid of such self-destructive burdens by denying the reality of their illness. But, of course, that is self-destructive in its own way. Others attempt to bury the baggage and its cargo of negativity by *pretending* that they are self-accepting, self-confident, and in control, even though they are not.

For some of us, the most effective way to lighten the load and rebuild self-worth is by turning again to God. We reaffirm our belief that He accepts and loves us exactly as we are right now.

If at times we see ourselves as limited in some way, we try to remember that in God's sight we are perfect. God loves us today as much as He did before we became ill. He will continue to love and support us no matter what changes take place in our health and our lives.

THOUGHT FOR TODAY

I am the same as ever; capable
of loving and worthy of love.

> "Create in me a clean heart, O God;
> and renew a right spirit within me."
>
> PSALMS 51:10

You can't remember the last time you had a meaningful conversation with your father. Your relationship with him has been severely strained for, what, ten years now? Even at family get-togethers you greet each other with barely discernible nods.

Now you are gravely ill. The cancer is very aggressive; you know it, and everyone else in the family does too. And for the first time in years your father is trying to reach out to you. To be completely honest, you have a tormenting ambivalence about the situation. You're ashamed of the side of you that wants to go on hating him; and you wish you could nurture the side that wants to rebuild the relationship.

So you try to put yourself in your father's shoes. How heart-wrenching it must be for him to stand by powerlessly as you are being dragged down by this catastrophic illness. And because the relationship is dysfunctional, his emotional pain must be all the more intense.

It's clear now that you can't run away and you can't let it slide by. That's not who you are or the way you choose to live. So you do your very best to appreciate his concern and accept his love and, at the same time, to be kind and loving to him.

THOUGHT FOR TODAY

The loving way is the right way.

"Look in my face: my name is Might-have-been;
I am also called No-more, Too-late, Farewell."

DANTE GABRIEL ROSSETTI

It seems unlikely that a severely strained relationship will be suddenly transformed in the face of grave illness because one of the people involved decides to reach out and let bygones be bygones. However, illness sometimes brings people together in spite of themselves.

These types of situations are opportunities to put spiritual principles into action, to try to practice unconditional love, for example. In that spirit, we reach out lovingly with no strings attached, without the expectation of a certain response or result.

How do we break through a long-standing barrier for the first time? The best way to express our feelings is simply, slowly, and with great clarity: "I know how sorry you are about my illness and that you care very deeply. Just knowing that brings me a great deal of comfort."

Following that, we can demonstrate our sincerity through encouraging gestures and actions. If we're still having trouble rebuilding the relationship, we can enlist a parent, brother, or sister to help make our feelings clear.

THOUGHT FOR TODAY

Love lives on.

March 12

> "Hope, that with honey
> blends the cup of pain."
>
> SIR WILLIAM JONES

Because my pain often attacks suddenly, it just as suddenly retreats, and then without warning roars back again; combating it requires as much guesswork as strategy. Even when my guesses are on target, the weapons I select from my pain-control arsenal—medication, meditation, or distraction—rarely eliminate the pain entirely but only temper it. To compound the challenge, what works well one day may not work at all the next.

Yet there's one approach I can always count on. When pain is raging and resistant, I'm better able to cope when I'm at my best emotionally. Having said that, I must quickly add that emotional strength doesn't come to me out of the blue. It requires cultivation, a willingness to focus on positive expectations rather than negative projections, and a shift in attitude and outlook from desperation to faith.

I'm healthiest emotionally, and thereby better able to transcend pain, when I have strong positive feelings toward others. The times I have feelings of love and appreciation for my friends and family members are the times I experience the deepest sense of well-being.

THOUGHT FOR TODAY

Can I focus less on the physical and more
on the emotional and spiritual?

> "Comparison, more than reality,
> makes man happy or wretched."
>
> THOMAS FULLER

You talk to a woman who had the same kind of cancer that you have. She was diagnosed and treated quickly and three months later her cancer was in remission; no surgery, no radiation. Your hopes soar and so do your expectations. Then you hear about someone else who was diagnosed in January and died in March. Your hopes vanish, your expectations turn wholly negative, and you fear that death is inevitable and imminent.

Obviously, comparisons of this sort are not in our best interest. The single most important factor in dealing with cancer or any other life-threatening illness is that *nothing is typical.*

Certainly, there is no typical patient; we all have different experiences. In the case of cancer, for example, there are not only many different forms, but also different levels. Symptoms also are different for each of us; so too are the preferred treatments and our responses to those treatments.

To be sure, we can learn a lot by listening to the experiences of others. However, it's essential that we do so objectively and with a degree of detachment; otherwise, we are likely to turn our open minds into closed ones.

THOUGHT FOR TODAY

I can't assume that my illness will behave and respond exactly like someone else's illness.

> "Honor a physician with the honor due unto
> him for the uses which ye may have of him:
> for the Lord hath created him."
>
> APOCRYPHA, ECCLESIASTICUS 38:1–3

My friend phoned me to vent her anger; when she was finished she said she felt better. Then she apologized, thanked me, and hung up. The focus of her fury was her oncologist, who had been insensitive and detached as he rushed her through a weekly checkup that morning. "I felt like one of fifty faceless patients passing through on a conveyor belt," she fumed.

We've all had similar experiences and feelings during visits to doctors. At one time or another, every one of us has been rushed, patronized, or treated disrespectfully. Following such episodes, it is tempting to conclude that physicians care less about medicine than they do about money and that the most important charts in their lives can be found in the financial sections of newspapers.

The truth is that few doctors choose their specialty purely for financial gain. Once we are over our annoyance at the slight we have experienced, can we really believe that any doctor can counsel hundreds upon hundreds of patients, many critically ill and some terminal, and remain unaffected by other people's pain?

THOUGHT FOR TODAY

Do I unfairly disparage all doctors
as "callous and greedy"?

"When the frustration of my helplessness
seemed greatest, I discovered God's grace
was more than sufficient."

CHARLES CALEB COLTON

Illness usually takes us by surprise, slipping into our lives like a thief in the night. Before we have a chance to regain our senses it can strip us of our carefree spirit, our dignity, our self-confidence, and as much as anything else, our once-strong sense of belonging.

Thieves always take and never give, so it's hard to imagine gaining anything from illness. Yet, over time, we have indeed gained at least one highly valuable asset, humility, which had always seemed well out of our reach.

In the past, many of us arrogantly believed that we would be healthy forever; self-centeredness convinced us that we were somehow immune to the realities of life. When illness brought us to our knees and showed us just how vulnerable we were, that's when we gained our first measure of humility. Only then was it possible for us to graciously ask for and gratefully accept help.

Illness also taught us to recognize and accept our powerlessness over people, places, and things. We became better able to see ourselves in perspective with others and the world as a whole. We gained a true sense of what is important and what is not.

THOUGHT FOR TODAY

Am I open to the lessons and
rewards of illness?

March 16

"Words are the dress of thoughts; which should
no more be presented in rags, tatters,
and dirt, than your person should."

PHILIP STANHOPE, LORD CHESTERFIELD

The words we use in conversations are often good indicators of certain prejudices or attitudes we may have, even though we may not be fully aware of them. If we blurt out to someone, for example, that we're "hobbling along like a cripple," then that statement reveals quite a lot about our self-image, not to mention our feelings about people (including ourselves) who may be physically challenged.

Similarly, if after two days and nights of unrelenting pain we tell our partner that we're going to "break down and call the doctor," that says much about our attitude toward healthcare professionals and also, very likely, about our level of self-worth.

What exactly do we mean when we say we're "going to break down and call the doctor?" Do we feel that it's somehow improper to interrupt the doctor with anything less than a dire emergency? Does our choice of words indicate we're afraid the doctor might be annoyed by one too many calls from us and that we don't want to risk disapproval? Do we feel that the doctor is too important to be bothered by the likes of us?

THOUGHT FOR TODAY

My words reflect my feelings. If I change
the feelings, the words will follow.

"Humility is to make a right
estimate of one's self."

CHARLES HADDON SPURGEON

I don't know how long it took me to regain consciousness following open-heart surgery, but I clearly remember how surprised and grateful I felt to be alive. For quite some time after that, perhaps a year or more, I had little trouble putting my spiritual beliefs into practice. I was quite willing to work for a full recovery and completely willing to leave the results to God.

Looking back, it seems that I gained a degree of humility from that near-death experience. I realized (not for the first time) that I wasn't in control of my world or anyone else's.

As time went on and I became stronger, my ego expanded along with my confidence. I frequently tried to take control in areas where I was completely powerless. The best I could do was rarely good enough; gradually self-will again became a damaging force in my life.

The more I tried to take control, the more fearful I became. I was humbled once more and realized I had forgotten this vital spiritual principle: By doing the best I can, and then surrendering the results to God, I allow His power to enter my life and bring about positive change.

THOUGHT FOR TODAY

God is in charge. If it is supposed
to happen, it will.

March 18

> "Recall your courage,
> and lay aside sad fear."
>
> VIRGIL

It goes without saying, doesn't it, that risk-taking no longer belongs in our lives? Risks are for healthy people who can still afford to put themselves on the line. These days we want to feel protected, not vulnerable; solid, not fragile; secure, not fearful. Now that we're sick and frequently in pain, risk-taking is the last thing in the world we should expect of ourselves. Right?

Wrong. The reality is that certain risks are well worth taking and, in fact, can bring comfort and even more security to our lives. We stand to benefit greatly, for example, when we risk becoming more self-aware by exploring our feelings and reactions, by learning to identify and eliminate old ideas and character flaws, and by practicing meditation.

Risks can also bring rewards when we share our emotions and personal experiences with friends and loved ones—when, by risking intimacy, we allow others to know us at the truly important levels instead of merely the superficial ones.

For many of us, the most beneficial risk of all is the one we take by letting go and letting God.

THOUGHT FOR TODAY

Before I automatically say no, I'll
check the risk-reward ratio.

"But the waiting time, my brothers,
Is the hardest time of all."
SARAH DOUDNEY

The worst thing about the biopsy is not the anesthetic, the probing, the suture removal, or the scarring. The worst thing, of course, is waiting for the results.

There have been other times, when you waited anxiously for word about a college application, a job assignment, or an offer on a house. But waiting for crucial medical results is in another league entirely. The outcome this time could overshadow and upend everything else in your life.

As difficult as it is to wait twenty-four hours, seventy-two hours, or even a week for test results and a definitive diagnosis, there are actions you can take to lighten the emotional burden. First of all, keep yourself as busy as possible. It doesn't matter what activities you choose, so long as they help divert your thoughts from fearful and negative projection. For the same reason, surround yourself with loving and caring friends and family members.

If you have faith in a Power greater than yourself and spirituality is important in your life, you already know what to do. You've learned that letting go and letting God is the one action, more than any other action, which will safely carry you through this trying time.

THOUGHT FOR TODAY

While I am waiting, I will prepare myself by
strengthening my emotional and spiritual resources.

March 20

> "I would not anticipate the relish of any happiness, nor feel the weight of any misery, before it actually arrives."
>
> JOSEPH ADDISON

A ray of sunlight at the edge of the window awakened me the other morning. As I watched it grow brighter, I cautiously arched my back and raised my arms. Instead of feeling the usual jolts of pain, I was surprisingly supple and relaxed.

I vowed to fully enjoy the unexpected period of pain-free grace for however long it might last. For the next several days I felt better than I had in months. I took the opportunity to enjoy activities that are usually beyond my capabilities. And I was grateful.

I used to react quite differently during temporary remissions. I would become elated, almost manic. Right away I would conclude that I had eluded and escaped pain once and for all, forever. Needless to say, my unrealistic expectations made the inevitable relapse seem much worse than it actually was.

Time after time I baited the trap and then sprung it on my own neck. It took numerous such episodes for me to finally realize how I had been setting myself up for those crushing disappointments. Now, I try to make the most of each day as it comes—not just the sunny ones, but the dreary ones too.

THOUGHT FOR TODAY

I will accept each new moment of grace, gratefully and gracefully.

"All things are what
you make them."

PLAUTUS

One of the first things we discover in support groups is that even though our illnesses may be similar, we tend to "wear" them in different ways. Some of us respond and react to chronic illness and pain with a great deal of negativity; we put ourselves through lengthy periods of despair and isolation. Others become bitter and angry at society, government, parents, doctors, or God. Still others, driven by fear, become cynical and hurtful.

On another level, many people work hard to become accepting of pain and illness and try to view the conditions as natural parts of life. Some look for spiritual meaning in illness; for them it becomes an opportunity for personal growth. Along the same lines, some see illness as a guidepost of sorts, a signal to unburden themselves of tormenting character traits. They become willing to let go of resentments, to be healed through forgiveness.

Each of us has the opportunity to choose how we "wear" the illness. And each day we can choose again and start anew.

THOUGHT FOR TODAY

I choose acceptance,
and life.

March 22

"God asks no man whether he will accept life.
That is not the choice. You *must* take it.
The only choice is *how*."

HENRY WARD BEECHER

The treatment process for just about every illness begins with attempts to discover and counteract a harmful organism, substance, deterioration, or malfunction that jeopardizes health or life. Then, once the initial crisis has passed, we may be motivated or even inspired to examine key areas of our life in the interest of continuing recovery and ultimate wellness. We do our best to make beneficial changes in our diet, work schedule, daily routine, and approach to stress.

But what about our relationships? We all know how painful and debilitating it is to be in discordant, unhealthy, or truly toxic relationships. With each traumatic turn of events or unsettling confrontation we feel alternately guilty, fearful, disappointed, confused, and exhausted.

This is not to suggest that we should automatically or ruthlessly eliminate toxic people from our life "in the interest of our health." However, we would do well to take a close look at all of our relationships in order to determine which ones are building us up and which are tearing us down. We can then decide which to nurture, which to put on hold, and which to end.

THOUGHT FOR TODAY

Now, more than ever, I must carefully
choose whom I allow into my life.

"Reason guides but a small part of man, and that
the least interesting. The rest obeys feeling,
true or false, and passion, good or bad."

JOSEPH ROUX

Until recently, we thought of ourselves as emotionally fragile. We were highly sensitive individuals, easily upset by difficult people and unexpected situations. Not surprisingly, the turmoil we created within ourselves was often far worse than the outside events that set us off.

But now, thankfully, we've begun to react and respond quite differently. We've learned that negative thoughts and feelings can harm us only if we allow them to do so. We've discovered that potentially destructive attitudes and reactions affect us only if we become attached to them. These days when we notice negative thoughts and ideas entering our mind, we let them flow through rather than dwell on them.

We have also found that we can calm our minds and emotions with spirituality. We have come to believe that God's peace can help us respond with equanimity and poise to events and circumstances that in the past would have caused us great distress.

We are still sensitive, positively so, but we have found ways to govern our thoughts and feelings and remain serene.

THOUGHT FOR TODAY

I own my feelings; they
do not own me.

March 24

> "Our chief want in life is somebody who
> shall make us do what we can."
>
> RALPH WALDO EMERSON

On the last day of your hospital stay the surgeon stood at the side of your bed and said, "Your inclination will be to let your wife do everything for you. But that will hurt you more than help you. You have to start doing things for yourself again; you have to rebuild your strength and self-worth."

You haven't yet found the ideal balance between doing too much and doing too little for yourself, but you are making progress. You're learning to accept help without hindering your recovery. You are also finding ways to make your wife and other loved ones feel important and needed, by showing that you value their company, opinions, and suggestions.

You've also discovered that the little things you're learning to do for yourself—giving yourself a sponge bath, airing out the room, preparing a sandwich—bring not only personal satisfaction but a real sense of recovery.

You are grateful now that the surgeon cautioned you. You no longer feel the need for constant pampering. Slowly but surely, you are achieving your goal of becoming as independent as possible.

THOUGHT FOR TODAY

Independence is within reach, one step
at a time, one day at a time.

"Pain is inevitable; suffering is optional."

BUDDHIST SPIRITUAL

I once watched a documentary on doctors who have cancer. The film showed how the doctors' personal experiences with the disease had brought about profound changes in their ability to understand and respond to patients' needs.

In an especially memorable segment of the film, one of the doctors took over the care of a terminally ill woman who had long been experiencing excruciating pain. The first thing the doctor did was to relieve her suffering by treating the pain adequately. During her previous treatment program the woman had lost the will to live because pain consumed every waking moment. As soon as her pain was compassionately treated, a dramatically positive transformation took place; her entire attitude and outlook changed.

She became able again to receive visitors and converse with her family, to give and receive love. She began to smile again, and even though she knew she was dying, she treasured each of her remaining days.

The film helped me realize clearly and powerfully how pain— especially treatable, *needless* pain—erodes the substance and quality of life. I have since asked myself, more than once, if my own pain is being treated empathetically, thoroughly, and properly.

THOUGHT FOR TODAY

Am I suffering needlessly?

March 26

"If you are distressed by anything external, the pain is not due to the thing itself but to your own estimate of it; and this you have the power to revoke at any moment."

MARCUS AURELIUS

Our bodies react to threatening or maddening situations in predictable ways. The heart pounds, breathing becomes rapid, muscles tense, and we also get that familiar butterfly feeling in our stomach. When such hormonal rushes occur, most of us allow ourselves to be swept away. We react angrily, or defensively, and later we pay the physical and emotional price.

In the interest of self-preservation we're learning how to remain grounded and centered in stressful situations. The key is to become aware, at the earliest possible moment, of emotional and physical indications of stress. If we're successful, at that point we can choose a constructive response instead of automatically reacting destructively.

For example, when our heart races, our palms sweat, and we begin to feel anxious, we can try to stabilize ourselves by focusing on deep, rhythmic breathing. Similarly, when our face reddens and we feel our shoulders tighten, we can calm ourselves with thoughts or words such as these: "I'm tensing up and I'm on the edge; but I don't have to go over."

It takes practice to become immediately aware of stress indicators as they begin to occur. It also takes discipline to *respond* constructively in new ways, rather than *react* destructively in the same old ways.

THOUGHT FOR TODAY

I've discovered a new area of control;
I can respond, rather than react.

> "Above all, keep loving one
> another earnestly...."
>
> THE GOSPEL OF PETER

Sexual intimacy allows us to express feelings of love and closeness in a very special way. Chronic illness may not necessarily reduce the desire and need for such intimacy, but it certainly can put it to the test. We may convince ourselves that sex is no longer enjoyable, important, or possible, and allow that aspect of our life to fade into the background.

Chronic illness can wreak havoc with self-image and self-esteem. We may feel unattractive, undesirable, and unworthy. And since our sexuality is closely linked with the way we feel about ourselves, this leads to confusion and mixed messages. For example, because of a poor self-image, we may send "keep away" signals even though we want our partner to draw closer. Or, because our partner thinks we need rest when in fact we desire sexual intimacy, he or she may become less assertive. So our sex life dwindles.

Chronic illness or not, we still need to love and be loved. We still desire the physical and emotional stimulus and release that sex provides. It is a mistake to pretend that sexuality and sex are no longer necessary and important when they truly are.

THOUGHT FOR TODAY

Physical intimacy can
enhance self-esteem.

March 28

"Talking is like playing on the harp; there is as much in laying the hand on the strings to stop their vibrations as in twanging them to bring out their music."

OLIVER WENDELL HOLMES

When sexual activity has diminished or disappeared because of the physical and emotional trauma of illness, what can we do to revitalize that special bond and, in the process, strengthen the relationship overall?

Communication—honest, loving, trusting communication—is without a doubt the essential first step. When we openly discuss this sensitive and often difficult subject with our partner, we are likely to learn a great deal about one another's feelings and concerns.

We may be surprised to discover that our partner misses sexual intimacy as much as we do. We may find that a frayed self-image has led to avoidance. We may be able to quickly unscramble mixed messages, patch up hurt feelings, and move forward together.

Communication of this sort can also open the door to practical considerations. For example, there may be a need for flexibility and experimentation in response to such physical aspects of chronic illness as pain, fatigue, or limited range of motion. It may turn out that where once spontaneity was a measure of mutual affection, the timing and planning are now more important factors in the equation.

THOUGHT FOR TODAY

We will talk, we will listen, and we will grow close again.

"He has made everything beautiful in its time;
also He has put eternity into man's mind."

ECCLESIASTES 3:11

Several years ago I traveled from the United States to Germany. It was mid-March, still quite cold and wet, the deciduous trees were bare, and little color could be seen anywhere. I was disappointed that winter had not yet loosened its grip.

Ten days or so into my trip, on a relatively warm Sunday, I was walking along the Lichtentaler Allee in Baden-Baden. When I stopped for a moment to look around, my breath caught in my throat. There was a light green haze on the tree branches; everywhere I looked, daffodils, jonquils, tulips, and hyacinths had begun to push upward through the dark soil. I realized at that moment that everything was coming to life right before my eyes and practically under my feet!

That night, I reflected about the excitement I had felt witnessing spring literally bursting forth. It struck me that there is always seasonality and the cycle of change; always transformation and renewal; always life. Even in the face of serious illness or probable death, we can be heartened, gladdened, and joyfully reconnected with nature and God for whatever journey lies ahead.

THOUGHT FOR TODAY

Perhaps the miracle is already
in process.

> "Self-confidence is the first requisite
> to great undertakings."
>
> SAMUEL JOHNSON

Some of us have parents who can best be described as controlling. They love us, that's a given; the problem is that they've attempted to run our lives for as far back as we can remember.

The problem has taken on a painful new dimension now that we're ill. Because our parents are so frustrated by their lack of control over our disease, they second-guess every decision large and small. Implying that we've made a series of dangerous mistakes, they question not only our choice of physician but also his or her diagnosis, treatment plan, and prescriptions.

We're already fragile and vulnerable because of the illness. The constant questioning and negativity only serve to undermine the foundation of confidence we've been trying to build.

What's the best way to deal with parents who constantly put us on the defensive and generate wave after wave of self-doubt? First, we decide in advance just how much information we're willing to share. Second, and more important, we respond to each barrage of questions promptly and assertively, along these lines: I appreciate your concern, I really do, but I have full confidence in my doctor and the treatment plan we've worked out together.

THOUGHT FOR TODAY

I can and will stand my ground.

"If the brain sows not corn,
it plants thistles."

GEORGE HERBERT

Your mind has taken you hostage; for hours now it has been torturing you. The jabs are white-hot and agonizing. They come at you in a relentless, screaming blur.

Will there be a scar on the outside? How big, how obvious? Is this real pain now, or am I imagining it? Will there be more pain later? How will I be able to stand it? This doctor, is he competent? Will there be blood transfusions? How safe? What will it all cost? Will they cancel my insurance?

These are just a few of the phantom concerns posed by your torturer. The real questions you need to answer are these: How can I escape my mind? How can I divert it? How can I regain control?

Focus on your breathing, the inhalations and exhalations. That way your mind will be fully occupied with something new, and it won't be able to torment you.

Visualize a symbol that means something special and direct your mind to that image. It could be a healing light, a wonder of nature, or your personal perception of God.

Recite a mantra, silently or aloud, to effectively drown out your mind's hurtful assaults. Set yourself free.

THOUGHT FOR TODAY

My mind can focus on only
one thing at a time.

April

"It is better to take many small steps in the
right direction than to make a great leap forward
only to stumble backward."

CHINESE PROVERB

Those of us who are cancer survivors learn to walk a fine line in certain areas of our new life. As one important example, we try to take the best possible care of ourselves without allowing the disease to become the centerpiece of our existence. In particular, we try to stay alert for signs of recurrence or new symptoms, without going overboard and creating an atmosphere of constant alarm.

In the past we were usually able to remain levelheaded in the face of threatening events or actual calamities. These days, though, it's difficult not to become frightened by physical changes that might foreshadow further problems. Yet we need not feel guilty about such apprehension; after all, we've already been to the edge.

Our doctors don't always seem to understand how difficult it is for us to walk that fine line between responsibility and panic. They have their own problems and occasionally are not sympathetic to our concerns. So it's up to us to explain, to let them know the kinds of feelings we're having and why we're having them. Following that, all we can do is try to let it go and continue doing what we know is right.

THOUGHT FOR TODAY

I will try to see each checkup as
health *care*, not health *crisis*.

April 2

"Health is not simply the
absence of sickness."

ANONYMOUS

When one of my brothers turned sixty, we threw him a surprise birthday party. Several dozen relatives, colleagues, and friends converged at his New England home. Traveling from the West Coast, I was the first to arrive.

The party lasted through the weekend. Although I joined in all the festivities, I made it a point to pace myself, to get plenty of rest, and also to enjoy the stillness of nearby woods. On the flight home I felt terrific; my brother had been surprised and thrilled, and my lupus had not been a problem.

Then I ruined it. As soon as I got home I plunged into frenetic activity. I fixed a broken door lock; caught up with a week's worth of mail, newspapers, and phone messages; did several loads of laundry; went to the market; and started back to work—all while suffering the effects of jet lag. Within forty-eight hours I had a major lupus flare-up.

I'd done the same thing to myself following other trips. You'd think I would have remembered how important it is for chronically ill people to take a few days to recover from travel before easing back into regular routines. Well, next time will be different.

THOUGHT FOR TODAY

I will respect my body's health needs.

> "Nothing is so firmly believed
> as what we least know."
>
> MICHEL EYQUEM DE MONTAIGNE

We understood very little about illness. Even when people close to us were afflicted, we distanced ourselves emotionally. Because of such avoidance, we had to overcome many misconceptions when we became ill ourselves.

We believed, for example, that illness diminished us, and that we would henceforth live a low-quality life. We felt that no one could possibly understand what we were going through. We were certain that the treatment recommended for our condition wouldn't work and, moreover, that it would debilitate us with side effects. One of the most unyielding threads in our fabric of mythology was the belief that we could do nothing to help ourselves and that only the actions of others were important.

We eventually realized that if we were to heal and go on living productive lives, we would have to give up such self-destructive misconceptions. We would have to become active and open-minded students, let go of old ideas, and search out new truths. Honestly and fearlessly, we would have to find answers to questions we once were afraid to ask.

THOUGHT FOR TODAY

My beliefs and attitudes shape
and color my experiences.

> "The strongest principle of
> growth lies in human choice."
>
> GEORGE ELIOT

We all know that illness can be tyrannical, confining, and, on occasion, even enslaving. Sometimes at night when our loved ones are asleep, we think back with longing to the days when we were entirely free. But then we reflect at a deeper level and remember with gratitude that we are as free now as ever, illness notwithstanding.

We are free to use the God-given gifts of mind and imagination to be entertained, enlightened, and transported.

We are free to make choices of infinite variety, from the promises we make and keep, to the way we approach each new day.

We are free from the past, capable of living comfortably and with positive purpose in the here and now. We have broken free of the restraints of resentment, self-destructive behavior, and guilt.

We are free from the bondage of self and no longer limited by self-centered thoughts, emotions, or motives. We are free to reach beyond ourselves and focus on the needs and aspirations of others.

We are free to seek out new opportunities to explore and experiment. We are free to change in order to become ever-more free.

THOUGHT FOR TODAY

I celebrate freedom of mind and spirit.

"The Divine Spirit does not reside
in any except the joyful heart."

THE TALMUD

Lingering illness tends to narrow one's field of view. All too often I lose sight of my spiritual self and focus entirely on my physical self. One painful symptom surfaces, then another; new symptoms merge with old, drawing more and more of my attention to my body. Soon my emotions follow. Each reactive or defensive feeling—fear, self-pity, anger—draws me farther from my spiritual core. Before long, all I can think about is me, myself, and I, orbiting obsessively in a self-centered little universe.

This is not to say that I should try to deny the reality of my physical self. A certain degree of self-concern is necessary; these days it's more important than ever to listen carefully to my body and to respect its messages. However, in the interest of healing and wholeness it is equally important to nurture my spiritual essence.

To regain perspective and achieve balance, I first must quiet my mind and rein in my emotions. Then, I think about some of the ways illness has helped me grow spiritually. I reflect on God in my life and the struggles He has brought me through. I affirm the good He has in store for me.

THOUGHT FOR TODAY

My body is hardly the whole of me.

April 6

> "We want people to feel with us
> more than to act with us."
>
> GEORGE ELIOT

Several months after my lupus was diagnosed, I realized that some people didn't know how to act when they were visiting me, especially when my illness was causing me great pain and difficulty. While most visits from friends brought me comfort and fulfillment, some left me feeling empty and angry. I wondered what is it that I really want from visitors? After much thought, this is what I decided:

I want to be shown empathy, not pity. I also want to be treated as I was before I became ill.

I want my illness to be discussed openly and directly rather than with allusion or in whispers.

I want friends and loved ones to continue asking about the disease; that way, I know they're not afraid of it.

I want to be offered as much help as possible. I welcome practical suggestions, but I don't want to be pressured with second-guessing or unsolicited medical advice.

I want to be included in conversations about the wider world beyond my illness, in order to feel more connected to that world. And I want to be touched, hugged, and kissed just as before.

THOUGHT FOR TODAY

If I don't know how I want to be treated,
how can I let others know how to treat me?

"Why should I feel lonely?
Is not our planet in the Milky Way?"
HENRY DAVID THOREAU

Some of us were social butterflies; some were wallflowers; some were loners. In our old lives, we couldn't have been more dissimilar when it came to interaction with others. But now that chronic illness has brought us together we've discovered that, regardless of our background, these days every one of us sometimes feels alienated, disconnected, and utterly alone.

By sharing our experience, strength, and hope, we're beginning to understand that our alienation is not caused by the rigors of illness nor the actions of others. Rather, it is of our own making. Some of us choose to withdraw physically from friends and loved ones; we close the blinds, unplug the phone, and become reclusive. Others withdraw emotionally; going through the motions of life but never really "there."

We can see now that such isolation damages us and jeopardizes our recovery. We're rediscovering the healing power of connectedness. From each other we're learning how emotionally and spiritually rewarding it is to feel deeply attached to another person, to nature, to our own inner selves, and to our Creator.

THOUGHT FOR TODAY

I will strengthen the bonds of friendship and free myself from the bondage of alienation.

April 8

> "My words fly up, my thoughts remain below.
> Words without thoughts never to heaven go."
>
> WILLIAM SHAKESPEARE

I recently read about a gravely ill eleven-year-old boy whose parents worried that the sick child had no real sense of what it meant to die. With his mother present, the boy's pediatric oncologist talked with him in order to discover his feelings about death.

At one point the boy told the doctor that he said a special prayer every night. Then, without prompting, he said the prayer aloud. It spoke of the child's immortal soul, and of God's abiding love for him. Most interesting to the doctor was the way the child listened intently to his own words. The doctor said, "I think when he listened to himself praying that was more important than what anyone could say to him about death."

After reading the article, I couldn't help wondering about my prayers. Do I actually listen to what I say? Or do I simply pray by rote? Do my prayers serve as a channel through which I can ultimately learn God's will for me?

When I pray these days, I sometimes think of that eleven-year-old boy. And then I try to pray as a child would, and listen more carefully to what I am saying to my Creator.

THOUGHT FOR TODAY

When I talk to God, am I not
talking to myself as well?

"Nothing is so burdensome
as a secret."

FRENCH PROVERB

We usually keep secrets in the interest of self-preservation. More often than not, however, our secrets harm us rather than help us. That was the case with a young friend of mine.

When she was diagnosed with multiple sclerosis, she tried to hide the illness and her equilibrium problems from everyone but her immediate family. She did her best to remain isolated in her apartment. When visits by certain people became unavoidable, she would hide her cane, try to stay seated, and cut the visit as short as possible by pleading fatigue. My friend recalls that "Afterwards, I was always tormented by the possibility that my charade hadn't been successful."

The fear that she would be "found out" kept her awake night after night. In fact, it was sleeplessness that precipitated her decision to finally tell people about her disease.

"I had stigmatized myself," my friend said, "And it was such an enormous relief to come clean. I'd been so afraid of what people would think and say." She added, "What I feared most was that they would feel sorry for me. The reality is that hardly anyone pities me. Most of my friends couldn't be more respectful and supportive."

THOUGHT FOR TODAY

Secrets lock doors—and minds.

April 10

> "If all be well with belly, feet, and sides,
> A king's estate no greater good provides."
>
> HORACE

For years we walk, obliviously, past an unusual, cat-shaped rock on the way to the mailbox. Then, one day, we suddenly notice it with surprise and even awe. We've all had such experiences; the simplest or most obvious things are the ones to which we pay the least attention.

Perhaps the same is true in the management of chronic illness. Don't we tend to overlook the little things, even the tried and true basics that can increase comfort, decrease pain and frustration, and make a real difference overall?

If your hands ache because they are stiff and cold, for example, why not wear a pair of warm gloves to solve the problem? And what about purchasing a comfortable pair of shoes, the custom-fitted kind that will enable you to walk more often and more easily?

In the same spirit, perhaps now is the time to finally buy a comfortable recliner, or a new mattress, instead of waiting for that "once in a lifetime" sale.

Certainly each of us can come up with our own examples. The point is, by doing absolutely all we can to promote healing and peace of mind, we can raise our self-esteem and enhance our sense of well-being.

THOUGHT FOR TODAY

What can I do right now to make myself calm and comfortable?

> "In a higher world it is otherwise;
> but here below to live is to change,
> and to be perfect is to have changed often."
>
> JOHN HENRY NEWMAN

Your husband has fallen asleep on the couch. After having seen you through another day of health-related difficulties, he is understandably exhausted. Because you're feeling afraid and lonely, you're tempted to wake him up. Instead, however, you decide to leaf through a photo album.

Two years ago, hard to believe that's all it was. There are the two of you rafting down the Rio Grande. And there's that bright red rental van with the skis on top that you drove through Europe. Oh yes, there you are on the catamaran; the sight of your once-strong body and eager smile brings tears to your eyes.

You pull yourself together, as you have so often during the past year. So many things are different now. Your illness has brought about dramatic changes not only in your activities together, but in the relationship itself.

But you are doing your best to accept the new realities. Because you can't enjoy each other as you did before, you are creating new activities and new ways of relating. And you are holding fast to the conviction that your life together can still be as rich and meaningful as ever.

THOUGHT FOR TODAY

Create change.

April 12

> "Life is a sweet and joyful thing for one who has some one to love and a pure conscience."
>
> COUNT LEV NIKOLAYEVICH TOLSTOY

I mentioned to my wife at breakfast one morning that pain had kept me up half the night. Perhaps it was my imagination, but it seemed that she was fighting back tears as I told her. I realized right then, as never before, that when I hurt physically she hurts emotionally.

So I decided to try to keep my pain to myself, in order to spare my wife the sense of helplessness and frustration that she can't help feeling each time I say something about new or recurring pain. But then, after remaining close-mouthed for a week or so, I could tell that she was bewildered by my sudden silence. I felt a growing distance between us.

I rethought my decision, reminding myself that honest and open communication had always been at the heart of our relationship. It would be unfair of me to arbitrarily and unilaterally establish new boundaries, especially about something with such a major impact on both of our lives.

I reminded myself, too, that there is an enormous difference between communicating something to another person and simply "dumping" on them out of self-pity.

THOUGHT FOR TODAY

I'll be honest and open on the bad days,
and no less so on the good ones.

"Do not overrate what you have received,
nor envy others. He who envies others
does not obtain peace of mind."

PRINCE GAUTAMA SIDDHARTA

When illness drags us down to rock-bottom levels, it's easy to become envious of people who are not ill. There they are, free of pain, feeling good, leading fun-filled lives, while we are confined to bed. When we compare their circumstances to ours, envy is an understandable reaction. There's no harm in it. Right?

Not really. Occasional envious feelings may be understandable, and we may even take a degree of comfort from them, but envy is truly one of the most damaging emotions we can indulge in.

For one thing, envy keeps us stirred up and even agitated. It breeds not only dissatisfaction but, even worse, the sense that we are somehow "less than" those we envy.

From a physiological standpoint, envy is a wholly negative emotion that can actually suppress the immune system and, over time, diminish the body's healing powers.

Strong and frequent feelings of envy also may indicate that we are having a problem with acceptance. Certainly this is a familiar challenge for those of us with chronic illness. As we all know, the greater our degree of acceptance, the more centered, serene, and comfortable we are.

THOUGHT FOR TODAY

Self-acceptance first eliminates the pain of
envy, and then removes its cause.

April 14

"The wounded body shrinks from
even a gentle touch; an empty shadow
fills the anxious with fear."

OVID

Illness almost always breeds fear, sometimes to the point where the fear becomes an illness itself. Fear of this sort can so distort reality that we become paralyzed. Fear of the unknown, for example, keeps us in denial about our disease. We refuse to acknowledge its impact on our lives and are unwilling to learn about treatment options.

Fear can imprison us. We may give up traveling out of fear that a relapse or flare-up of our illness will leave us incapacitated, stranded, and forgotten.

We may become so ashamed and confused by illness-related fears that we feel they are too painful to discuss with others. Behavior of this kind not only isolates us but also can damage treasured relationships.

The fears we face today may seem more challenging than any in the past. That is the nature of fear; it *always* seems overwhelming. Yet with willingness, effort, and faith, it can *always* be overcome.

THOUGHT FOR TODAY
Fear may shield me from reality,
but it is not my friend.

"Just as courage imperils life,
fear protects it."

LEONARDO DA VINCI

We've known for a long time that illness is often accompanied by fear, and we've learned what happens when we try to ignore or bury that fear. It mushrooms, then suffocates and tyrannizes us so that our world becomes smaller and ever-smaller.

Thankfully, we have a strong and clear-cut choice. Instead of being at the mercy of our fears, we can channel fear-generated emotions into positive actions. Indeed, fear can be a powerful, life-enhancing motivator.

As an important example, our anxieties about a possible future cancer recurrence, lupus flare-up, or brain-damaging blood clot can motivate us to take far better care of ourselves, not only physically, but also emotionally, and spiritually. Fear can motivate us to eat properly, exercise regularly, and rest more. It can also lead us into stress-reducing activities such as meditation.

In the past, most of us have experienced fear as wholly negative and destructive. These days, however, we are learning that this potent emotion can frequently be used to our benefit.

THOUGHT FOR TODAY

Fear can tyrannize or motivate me;
the choice is mine.

April 16

There's that nurse again, the one who is so kind. It's such a pleasure to watch her work, to see the reactions of her patients as she takes care of them. For a moment or two their pain lines disappear; hostility melts away and frowns give way to smiles. She is our nurse, too, and whenever she enters the ward, we are up-lifted.

One day, last week, we had a revelation about our special nurse. We suddenly understood that her gentle ways and kindliness bring as much joy to her life as to the lives of others. The patients benefit greatly from her attention, there's no question about that. But it's clear now that she's receiving the richest rewards.

Perhaps we can follow her example. Perhaps we can rearrange our priorities and put kindness higher on the agenda. Starting right now, let's try to pass along the same sort of thoughtful and considerate words and actions we've appreciated receiving ourselves. Let's try to make a difference in the lives of others, and we too may be rewarded with feelings of joy and a sense of well-being.

THOUGHT FOR TODAY

I will reach out to you with loving
kindness, and help us both.

"Our life is a flying shadow, God the pole,
The needle pointing to Him is our soul."
ANONYMOUS

When a newscaster concluded his commentary the other night by saying, "So much has changed, so much has not," I took it personally. I thought, "Yes, that's exactly right."

Illness-related changes have affected many areas of my life, and while these changes are to be expected, they are nevertheless unsettling at times. I've had to drastically alter my work habits. My personal expectations and life goals are far different than before. And there have been major changes in the structure and content of my daily activities.

So much has changed, but then again, as the newscaster reminded me, so much has not. I can be comforted by remembering that I am still the same person, with the same personality and values. I can be warmed by the awareness that friends and loved ones still care about me and respect me as before.

Unchanged, too, is the spiritual core that grounds and sustains me. I still have and always will have the ability to put my spiritual principles into practice, to be kind, loving, and giving.

THOUGHT FOR TODAY

The winds of change are not always violent and destructive. At times they are gentle and favorable.

> "Patience and the mulberry leaf
> become a silk gown."
>
> CHINESE PROVERB

It's easy to become impatient when a five-minute delay stretches into an hour-long wait, when our expectations aren't met, or when things don't work out in accordance with our desires and designs. The problem, of course, is that impatience leads to stress, anger, discouragement, and self-pity. Impatience causes us to say and do things we later regret or to impulsively abandon important objectives and even necessary medical treatments.

Perhaps it's time to give some serious thought to the value of *patience*. When we cultivate patience we are able to think clearly, to make sound decisions, and to use our faculties to their best advantage. Patience allows us to maintain our composure and to feel confident and centered, whether we are faced with a minor frustration or a major crisis.

Patience brings with it a positive attitude and, very often, the willingness to be understanding, tolerant, and forgiving. By choosing patience over impatience—calmly doing what we can, then letting go and allowing things to work themselves out—we can more effectively solve problems while maintaining a sense of well-being.

THOUGHT FOR TODAY

Patience brings with it
dignity and self-respect.

"Now I am beginning to live a little, and feel
less like a sick oyster at low tide."

LOUISA MAY ALCOTT

Hospitals have a special energy, which can be both reassuring and distressing. Regardless of location or layout, they all seem to have the same sounds and smells, as well as a predictable pace of activity at different times of the day and night.

Those of us who have been hospital patients—who have been jostled on gurneys, draped and swabbed for surgery, or confined to noisy wards—rarely have fond memories of the stay. We associate hospitals with some of the very worst experiences of our lives.

Even in recovery, some of us dread going back for checkups or treatment. The wheelchairs and oversized elevators, the loudspeakers and surgical garb all bring us sharply back to a time we'd rather forget.

But we walk through the doors anyway. We grit our teeth when we sign in at the outpatient desk and then find our way to the lab or radiology department. We remind ourselves that these visits are essential to our continued well-being, and that it was in this very hospital that our lives were saved.

THOUGHT FOR TODAY

Putting distractions and painful memories
aside, I will focus solely on healing.

April 20

"It is always thus, impelled by a state of mind
which is destined not to last, that we make
our irrevocable decisions."

MARCEL PROUST

It's tough trying to decide whether or not to keep a job after you've become ill. At first, fear, uncertainty, and even self-consciousness can tempt you to act abruptly, to just go ahead and quit. However, staying on the job can work wonders for your self-esteem and sense of well-being.

Certainly the decision requires careful consideration and perhaps consultation with professionals. Ultimately, it depends on how you feel from day to day, on your attitude toward your illness and the job, and of course on your employer.

The first step is to talk to your employer or supervisor with complete candor. Be honest about your limitations, including the possibility that you may miss work occasionally. Talk about the need for rest breaks and modifications in your work area, if such considerations apply. Let your employer know what it will take for you to continue performing at a high level.

And remember: Good employees are hard to find and expensive to replace. So it's more than likely that your employer will be on your side.

THOUGHT FOR TODAY

When I'm faced with a life-affecting decision,
I'll take all the time I need.

> "It is an absolute perfection to know how to get
> the very most out of one's own individuality."
>
> MICHEL EYQUEM DE MONTAIGNE

We've all heard the expression "perfect patient." When illness strikes some of us try to be just that—the "perfect patient." Almost immediately, our unconscious minds burden us with expectations of how we should feel, how we should behave, and even how quickly we should heal.

Perhaps we had parents who, when sick, were stoic and uncomplaining to the point of denial. So we expect no less from ourselves. When we can't keep up the front—when self-pity and negative projection overflow—our "failure" adds guilt to the burden.

Some of us grew up with role models who claimed they never were sick a day in their life. They played off that fact by drumming into our heads the notion that "if you live right you'll stay healthy." Naturally, we feel that it's our own fault when we become ill.

Before we can move forward on the path to healing and wholeness, we must smash the myth of the "perfect patient." We must unchain ourselves from old ideas and outdated expectations and create our own expectations. By doing so, we give ourselves the opportunity to move toward wellness in our own unique way.

THOUGHT FOR TODAY

Trying to live up to someone else's
expectations is one burden too many.

April 22

> "What is without periods
> of rest will not endure."
>
> OVID

We rarely thought about or needed a rest during the day. When we wanted to "take a load off our feet," we would grab a cup of coffee or plop down in front of the TV and that would do the job.

These days, resting is far more than a catch-as-catch-can endeavor. It's as necessary to our well-being as food, water, medicine, and sleep. And it requires a certain amount of planning and preparation.

Our objective is to relax completely in order to become revitalized psychologically as well as physically. For most of us, the best way to accomplish this is to lie down, paying close attention to any pain or discomfort and adjusting our position accordingly.

We relax not only the body but also the mind, doing our best to ignore distracting thoughts. This is not a time to plan the remainder of the day or to figure out the solution to a puzzling problem.

Of course, how and where we rest needs to be tailored to our individual condition and circumstances. Whatever the case, *total relaxation* of mind and muscles for even a short period of time leads to a true sense of revitalization.

THOUGHT FOR TODAY

Though it may seem like a contradiction
in terms, rest is an important activity.

> "Pain is perfect misery, the worst
> Of evils, and excessive, overturns
> All patience."
>
> JOHN MILTON

My chronic pain is not constant, thank God for that. Each day there are windows of time when I am relatively pain-free. During those periods of grace, I try to take care of my responsibilities and participate in enjoyable activities.

To take advantage of such a pain-free afternoon recently, my wife and I packed a lunch and walked down to the beach. For an hour or so I was fine. Then, a fierce onslaught of pain practically brought me to tears.

My muscles tensed and my jaws clenched. My mood darkened and I became irritable. I complained about noisy seagulls and "outsiders" on the beach; I criticized my wife. When she responded by smiling and nodding her head knowingly, I realized what was happening: Severe pain had once again brought about a dramatic change in my attitude and behavior.

Whenever that happens I need to remind myself that I don't behave badly out of boorishness or malice; irritability is sometimes an unavoidable part of the pain package. However, that doesn't mean I should allow it to run its course unbridled, or that I myself have the right to run roughshod over others.

THOUGHT FOR TODAY

Although pain sometimes has a life of its own,
I won't let it take over my life.

April 24

> "Tears fall, no matter how we try to check them,
> and by being shed they ease the soul."
>
> SENECA

We've shed more tears in the last few months than in all the years of our lives, or so it seems. We've cried most often when alone, or late at night when everyone else in the family was sleeping. Occasionally, we've cried in front of other people—literally *bursting* into tears—and immediately felt foolish and embarrassed.

It's nonsense to feel embarrassed about crying, we know that, and we're trying to rise above the conditioning that tells us it's wrong to reveal our feelings in this manner. So when tears well up and we reflexively try to hold them back, we now do our best to override that reflex. We grant ourselves the freedom to cry; no matter who is nearby.

Crying is a natural and effective way of relieving tension. It's also a uniquely expressive way of letting others know the depth of our feelings and our needs.

Crying in the presence of others shows that we are willing to be vulnerable, to be known intimately. It also indicates that we are fully open to healing, whether it comes in the form of laughter, tears, or meditative silence.

THOUGHT FOR TODAY

Every one of my feelings is acceptable.

"Everything in life that we really
accept undergoes a change."
KATHERINE MANSFIELD

The doctors and counselors began talking about "acceptance" as soon as the diagnosis was definitive. Learning to practice acceptance would help us to heal and live peacefully, they said; acceptance would make it possible to channel our energy in positive directions rather than waste it by denying and resisting the disease.

For some of us the idea of accepting a debilitating and life-threatening illness was not only *un*acceptable, but unthinkable. We hated what the illness was doing to us and our families, and we'd be damned if we'd go down without a struggle.

That was our first reaction. Over time we've come to realize that acceptance doesn't mean we have to like or approve of what is happening in our life. Nor does it mean that we must passively resign ourselves to our "fate" and that we must give up our efforts to change and grow.

Acceptance is simply a willingness to see things as they really are, without being overwhelmed by that reality. Only then can we know what actions to take. Only then can we move forward with a clear-eyed view rather than continue to mark time in blind struggle.

THOUGHT FOR TODAY

Acceptance is not life-demeaning or
life-diminishing, but life-enhancing.

> ## "To forgive is beautiful."
> PUBLILIUS SYRUS

You know from experience that forgiveness is the antidote to resentment and is therefore one of the most healing actions you can take. You want to forgive one or more people, perhaps yourself as well, but you're finding it difficult to do so. Indeed, it's hard to even muster up the willingness.

Perhaps you feel that by forgiving someone you "give in" to that person's wrongful behavior and compromise your own dignity. Or you may feel that by withholding forgiveness you maintain an "edge" over those who wronged you.

It can be extremely useful at such times to apply what has been called the Divine Standard. Begin by focusing on God as you understand Him. Reflect on the nature of God's unconditional love for you and His willingness to be forgiving *no matter what* you may have said or done.

Ask yourself: Is God's love and forgiveness for past wrongs contingent on my present and future behavior? Is He impatient or judgmental of me or does He patiently accept me exactly as I am?

It goes without saying that none of us can achieve God's ability to love and forgive unconditionally. However, we can certainly try to emulate His Divine Standard.

THOUGHT FOR TODAY

I will try to forgive others and myself as God forgives— without contingencies or limitations.

> "We are so fond of one another,
> because our ailments are the same."
>
> JONATHAN SWIFT

As a cancer survivor, I'm involved with a support group called the Wellness Community. People like myself are encouraged to write their names, phone numbers, and brief cancer histories on index cards, which are placed in a red "Buddy Box." Newcomers to the Wellness Community use the box to contact people who have had the same type of cancer. My card is filed under Malignant Melanoma.

Several times a year I get a phone call from someone who has been newly diagnosed or who has had a recurrence. The person usually starts out by talking about doctors, hospitals, tests, and treatments. I try to steer the conversation toward the feelings and fears the caller is having and the effect the illness is having on his or her life.

Afterward, I always wonder if I've been at all helpful. It's hard to know. The thing is that I am able to listen empathetically; I understand what they're going through, because I've been there myself. Most of all, I think I'm able to offer hope. After all, I am a survivor. My cancer was diagnosed and surgically removed in 1981 and I'm cancer-free to this day.

THOUGHT FOR TODAY

Let's stick together;
let's keep hope alive.

April 28

> "Self-love, my liege, is not so vile a sin
> As self-neglecting."
>
> WILLIAM SHAKESPEARE

When we are called upon to take care of someone, our own experience with illness can be invaluable. We know what it's like to be challenged by pain, to have to follow a complex schedule of medications, and to depend on others for bathing, meals, and comforting.

It's wonderful to be able to give back what we were given during the difficult times of our own illness. On a deeper, spiritual level, the ability to now share our experience, strength, and hope gives real meaning and purpose to what we've been through.

However, there is a potential problem for us in certain care giving situations, especially those requiring long-term commitment on our part. We may get so caught up in the day to day, hour by hour needs of someone else that we forget about our own priorities. We may push ourselves too far, failing to eat right, to get enough rest, or to take time for self-renewal.

In order to be at our best we must look after our own physical, emotional, and spiritual needs. We should remember to treat ourselves with the same attentiveness and loving kindness with which we treat the patient.

THOUGHT FOR TODAY

Am I remembering the priorities
of my own health and well-being?

"Here is the place where the road
divides into two parts."

VIRGIL

It used to be that people who became seriously ill would take the arduous ride passively, with little foreknowledge of the route, or even the hoped-for destination. We've since realized that of all our choices, passivity is the worst one we can make. So we've begun to insist on a loud say concerning every aspect of the journey to wellness, and we're unwilling to leave the driving to others.

These days we prepare for our journey with road maps in the form of books, articles, and newsletters, plus any other information that can help us make decisions about our health care. We also join support groups, involving ourselves with others who already have been where we are going.

While we try not to lock horns with doctors who are accustomed to being in complete charge, we make it clear that we want to help plan our own treatment and care. We expect doctors and other healthcare professionals to share all relevant information with us, to spell out not only expected benefits but also possible risks from different treatments, and to treat us with the courtesy, honesty, and respect we deserve.

THOUGHT FOR TODAY

On this team, the only one who
can sideline me is me.

April 30

"Know then, whatever cheerful and serene,
supports the mind, supports the body too;
Hence, the most vital movement mortals feel Is hope,
the balm and lifeblood of the soul."

JOHN ARMSTRONG

Many of us have been in life-altering situations where we are encouraged by friends, family members, or healthcare professionals to keep hope alive. Often the phrase is spoken with little forethought; at times, it flows from deeply held conviction.

What do we really know about hope? Does the fact that we do or do not feel hopeful have any real influence on the course and eventual outcome of an illness? Is hope—as some cynics believe—a form of sophistry that shields us from reality?

My own experience over the years has led me to believe that it is always better to choose hope over resignation, even when no such choice has been presented or is evident. Hope is always well worth nurturing, if for no other reason than to temper fear and uncertainty.

There's no question in my mind that the positive messages inherent in hope, as opposed to those negative ones inherent in despair, can only serve to enhance my immune system. Hope helps me to heal and contributes greatly to my overall sense of well-being.

THOUGHT FOR TODAY

Hope is the high road.

May

May 1

> "Harmony is one phase of the law
> whose spiritual expression is love."
>
> JAMES ALLEN

Dinner needs to be cooked, but neither of you is well enough. Besides, the refrigerator is practically empty. You both need clean clothes and towels, but no one has the energy or capability to do the laundry.

It's hard enough for a healthy person to run a household and also care for a partner who is ill, but the challenge can seem overwhelming when both people are sick. At such times, it's tempting to commiserate together, to feed off each other's suffering, and even to wallow in mutual self-pity.

As some of us have learned from painful experience, such attitudes and behavior only serve to exacerbate the illnesses, and also to magnify any stresses that existed in the relationship before illness struck. At first, we empathetically compare symptoms with each other; before long, the dynamics of the relationship change and we are at each other's throats.

In such complex and difficult situations, consideration, tolerance, and sensitivity—at the very least—must become the order of each day. Beyond that, a flexible plan can be (*needs* to be) worked out and implemented in order to meet the challenge.

THOUGHT FOR TODAY

We can bring healing and harmony
out of chaos and conflict.

> "All experience is an arch,
> to build upon."
>
> HENRY ADAMS

Life can quickly turn chaotic when both of you are ill at the same time. However, you need not throw up your hands, for there are solutions. Obviously, pragmatic challenges such as cooking, cleaning, and marketing have to be managed, perhaps with the assistance of friends, relatives, or neighbors. No less important, however, are the emotional and spiritual aspects of the situation. Here are some suggestions to make it easier for you and your partner to live in harmony while helping each other heal.

Agree at the outset—make a "pact"—to be extra thoughtful, attentive, and loving to each other, one day at a time. Recognize the need for each of you to have time alone.

Try not to complain too much, not only for your own sake, but also to avoid dragging your partner down with you. If you must complain, try to balance your litany of miseries with possible solutions. Along the same lines, talk about blessings you share.

Whenever possible (or desirable), participate together in such wellness activities as meditation, stretching, and creative visualization. Last, but certainly not least, make plans for one or more "fun activities" you can look forward to when you are both feeling better.

THOUGHT FOR TODAY

Bridges, not barriers.

May 3

"Death with the might of his sunbeam,
Touches the flesh, and the soul awakes."

ROBERT BROWNING

When it became clear that my father's cancer was terminal and that he would soon die, I traveled to Florida to be with him. During the first week of my stay he was quite agitated and fearful. Then, a few days before his death, he became suddenly tranquil.

At one point my father suggested that I "bring coffee" to his mother, father, brothers, and sister, all of whom were apparently there in the room with him, even though they had died many years earlier. I understood then why he had become so peaceful. He was being lovingly drawn away from this world and the physical and emotional pain he had endured for so long.

The experience gave me a profound sense of peace and security that remains with me to this day. Like most people, I had often wondered fearfully about death: *Does it hurt? Do you just fade away? Is there a heaven, hell, and limbo? Do you see a light? Is it God? Do you come back in another form?*

I no longer need to know the answers to such questions. By witnessing the gentle nature of my father's peaceful passing, I learned that all I have to do is trust God.

THOUGHT FOR TODAY

When death comes,
God will continue caring for me.

"Better a blush on the cheek
than a spot in the heart."
MIGUEL DE CERVANTES SAAVEDRA

You are a very private person. Although you are not overly modest, you always have been somewhat reserved about your body; you're not a person who enjoys massages, facials, or even manicures. During recent months, however, your body has been probed, jabbed, manipulated, exposed, and discussed over-and-over-and-over again. You're at the point where even the prospect of a flimsy hospital gown and the chill of steel on your bare thighs is enough to send you screaming for cover.

You are angry, of course you are. You feel that your personal space is being violated and that your dignity is being compromised. Such feelings are certainly understandable; many of us react in exactly the same way.

The thing is, although there's a lot about healthcare and medical treatment we hate, we become willing to go through it anyway. It is somewhat easier to push modesty and self-consciousness aside when we acknowledge that our lives are at stake.

There's also this to consider: No matter how often or how painfully our bodies are prodded and probed, our souls and inner spirits—the essence of who we *truly* are—remain inviolable.

THOUGHT FOR TODAY

It's worth it.

> "Kick away the ladder,
> and one's feet are left dangling."
>
> MALAY PROVERB

Even when we were healthy, some of us hated to ask for help. We took pride in being self-sufficient, low-maintenance individuals, "who would rather do it myself, thank you very much." To this day, even when we clearly need help, we have trouble asking for it.

What accounts for our reluctance? For one thing, we may be unwilling to give up our image of health and independence. Also, we may be afraid of appearing too self-involved. Perhaps we don't want to let on how sick we really are. Or we may feel that we are burdens and that all we do is take, take, take.

Isn't it true, though, that our lives become even more difficult when we don't learn to reach out for help and accept it graciously?

The next time it's necessary to ask for assistance, let's think back to all the times we helped others. Let's remind ourselves, moreover, that even as we accept help today we can find new ways to reciprocate. We can share our experiences, adventures, strength, courage, and hope. We can connect with our helpers spiritually and intellectually and in the process enrich all of our lives.

THOUGHT FOR TODAY

Accepting help doesn't
make me helpless.

"There are no days in life so memorable, as those which vibrated to some stroke of the imagination."

RALPH WALDO EMERSON

As children, one of our most liberating discoveries was our imagination; when we were bored or in pain, we learned to transport ourselves to new realities, to more exciting and acceptable worlds.

Our imaginations have matured and we have learned to use them more productively and with greater versatility. Although the how, where, and why of imagination remains a mystery, we do believe that this wondrous faculty is a precious gift from God.

At times our imagination floods us with joyful expectations; on other occasions it shadows our world with foreboding. Fortunately, we are not wholly at the mercy of imagination. We can control and channel it to our advantage, as we did when we were young.

If a loved one is somewhat distant or inattentive today, how will we use our imagination? Will we paint images of loveless fury and create scenarios of abandonment? Or will we use our imagination to bring us back to reality, to understanding, and peace of mind?

If pain strikes or lingers, will we envision disaster and strike terror in our own hearts? Or will we, through positive imagining, infuse the afflicted area with healing light?

THOUGHT FOR TODAY

My imagination can free me.

"Manhood begins when we have in any way made truce with Necessity; begins even when we have surrendered to Necessity, as the most part only do; but begins joyfully and hopefully only when we have reconciled ourselves to Necessity; and thus, in reality, triumphed over it, and felt that in Necessity we are free."

THOMAS CARLYLE

Sometimes we are tempted—in fact, *compelled*—to disregard an illness and the physical limitations caused by it. This usually happens during the initial days or weeks following a diagnosis, when we are still in denial and not yet ready to acknowledge the seriousness of our condition.

Stubbornly and with fierce determination, we grit our teeth against the pain and plunge forward with activities that once were routine for us, but are now clearly beyond our capabilities: a high-powered game of racquetball, a twelve-hour workday, or a weekend of house painting. And, of course, we pay a heavy price.

Perhaps we have to go through such episodes in order to surrender to the reality of the illness. Eventually we do surrender, and little by little we learn to live fully and gracefully within the new framework of our life.

As time goes by and we become more skillful at practicing what has been called "the fine art of accommodation," we begin to understand a life-altering truth: Only by surrendering and accepting our limitations can we discover new capabilities and new opportunities.

THOUGHT FOR TODAY

Surrender does not confine me, but frees me.

"Tension is who you think you should be.
Relaxation is who you are."

CHINESE PROVERB

I read everything I can find on pain management and I occasionally attend lectures on the subject. It's comforting to know that healthcare professionals have begun to better understand that their patients' pain *needs* to be controlled and *can* be controlled.

It's also comforting to realize that I need not rely solely on my doctors' prescriptions for pain relief, and that I can do much on my own. Indeed, I often have the feeling that the ultimate responsibility is mine.

I have learned, as a primary example, that stress and muscle tension invariably worsen any pain I may be experiencing. On the other hand, when I'm relaxed and relatively free of stress, it's far easier to deal with my pain.

When I feel stress mounting and pain sharpening, here are some of the on-the-spot techniques I use to regain peace of mind and obtain relief. I take a short walk; I slow my mind by focusing on my breathing; I say the Serenity Prayer; I put my problems back in perspective by asking myself, "So what if . . . ?" "How important is it . . . ?" I visualize myself in a tranquil and pleasurable environment. I remind myself that God is in charge.

THOUGHT FOR TODAY

Less stress equals less pain.

May 9

> "Certain thoughts are prayers.
> There are moments when, whatever be the
> attitude of the body, the soul is on its knees."
>
> VICTOR HUGO

When we were very young, eight or nine years old, someone in our family became very ill. "Pray for her," we were told, and we did so, fiercely and repeatedly, for weeks. When she died we felt guilty because obviously we hadn't prayed hard enough, or long enough, or properly.

Our attitudes about prayer have changed a lot since then. When we pray these days it is with the conviction that in many areas of life we are powerless, while God has all power. We pray not so much for specific answers or outcomes, but with faith that Divine good will prevail.

As children we begged God to prolong the life of a loved one or to fulfill one or another of our deep desires. Today we pray not for personal fulfillment or gain, but to strengthen our partnership with God. If we have a specific objective, it is that His will be done.

The purpose of prayer is not to burden us, but to relieve us of our burdens. We pray in the spirit of letting go and letting God, and as a result we are finding freedom and inner peace.

THOUGHT FOR TODAY

Thy will be done.

"What can a sick man say, but that he is sick?"
SAMUEL JOHNSON

There aren't very many of them, but you know who they are, and you really don't appreciate their speculations about your illness. They are the well-meaning ones, even the loved ones and sometimes, in whispered innuendoes, and at other times boldly and straightforwardly, they point to such factors as stress, your ambitious nature, unresolved childhood issues, or bottled-up emotions as causes for the disease that has put your life in jeopardy. In short, they blame *you* for your illness, and that's cruel and hurtful.

The possible causes of your illness are none of their business, especially when they base their opinions on speculation and flimsy assumptions. The most harmful aspect of placing blame is that it diverts your attention to the past, when now more than ever you need to direct all of your energies to the present.

Why do they dig for "causes"? It's probably more out of ignorance than insensitivity. Perhaps to help themselves cope with the frightening reality of a life-threatening condition. Or, in order to understand and explain the illness, so they can convince themselves that the same thing won't happen to them.

In any case, the last things seriously ill people need are self-doubt, self-blame, and self-condemnation. What they do need, more than anything, is acceptance.

THOUGHT FOR TODAY

No one is to blame for my illness.

> "The sun shines and warms and lights us and we have no curiosity to know why this is so; but we ask the reason of all evil, of pain, and hunger, and mosquitoes and silly people."
>
> RALPH WALDO EMERSON

Occasionally we read something that has a profound impact on our lives. It may not be an entire book or article; it can be a single phrase or sentence that reaches deep inside of us and, for years thereafter, resonates.

That's what happened to me when I came across a statement by the late tennis star and humanitarian Arthur Ashe who asks, in his autobiography, "Why me?" The profundity of the question was buried deep in the book, *Days of Grace,* but it leaped out at me.

Like most people who suffer with chronic illness, as Ashe did, with AIDS, I can't help wondering occasionally, "Why me?" The thought is more likely to insinuate its way into my consciousness when pain has clouded my mind and weakened my faith. However, since reading Ashe's wise and challenging words, I've become better able to counteract my self-pity. I try to ask the same question, "Why me?" I ask it and think about all of the blessings in my life, past and present.

I live in a heated house and have plenty of food and the best medical care. *Why me?*

I am a fortunate man with the ability to earn a decent living. *Why me?*

My life is filled with loving relationships. *Why me?*

THOUGHT FOR TODAY

Let's think about the blessings.

"What I am to fear, I know not—
Yet none the less I fear all things."
OVID

It's easy to become preoccupied and even obsessed with our illnesses and the way they are affecting our bodies. Our temperature drops down to normal, but we worry that it won't stay that way, so we take it again ten minutes later, and then again half an hour after that. We've had the impression that we are "sensing" the world differently than usual, so we begin to scrutinize the way things around us look, taste, smell, and feel. We analyze the slightest fluctuation in our level of pain, and then speculate endlessly.

But our concerns are understandable, aren't they? After all, we so desperately want to feel better. And it's important to remain aware, isn't it?

Yes, we certainly want to get well, and yes, we must remain aware, but that doesn't mean we should go to extremes. When we obsessively analyze each real and imagined symptom, we create tremendous stress, not just for ourselves, but for everyone around us.

So let's try to achieve a balance between the two extremes of denial and preoccupation. Let's do our best to heal, but let's also allow it to happen.

THOUGHT FOR TODAY

Is my preoccupation with illness
shutting out the larger world?

May 13

> "Being in a good frame of mind helps keep
> one in the picture of health."
>
> ANONYMOUS

One of the most enjoyable things about traveling, even in one's own city, is "people-watching." We don't have to actually meet people; we can learn a great deal about them by the way they hold themselves and their body language.

That man, slouching forward and staring at the sidewalk, seems to have the weight of the world on his shoulders. That woman, her smiling face tilted upward and her stride purposeful and energetic, is joyful and on top of the world. That child—her body drawn inward and her eyes darting—seems utterly insecure and fearful.

What about our body language? How do we hold ourselves? Since our posture not only reflects but also *affects* our mental and emotional state, it is important to remain aware of our physical orientation, facial expressions, and any muscular tension.

Although it may seem simplistic, the reality is that our sense of well-being and, indeed, our actual self-esteem can improve as our posture improves. The taller and straighter we carry ourselves, and the more frequently we smile and relax our muscles, the better we feel, physically, mentally, and emotionally.

THOUGHT FOR TODAY

The way I carry myself says a lot
about my view of myself.

> "Sickness comes on horseback,
> but goes away on foot."
>
> WILLIAM CAREW HAZLITT

We've done it again. We've skipped taking two of our medications, and decided it's too late to take the third. Also, this makes twice in a row we've canceled our physical therapy appointment. And now we feel guilty for letting ourselves down.

Why, on some days, do we fail or even refuse to comply with our prescribed treatment program? Why do we prolong our suffering, or even risk a relapse?

We rationalize, "These pills are way too expensive to take so often." We focus on previous medications that "didn't work" and conclude that the new ones will be just as ineffective. We decide that we're too busy to meditate.

On a particular day, moreover, we may slide into denial, refusing to acknowledge or deal with our illness in any way. Or, we may make a misguided and futile decision to "take control." Finally, at an unconscious level, we may conclude we're not worthy of all the time and attention required by our illness.

One good way to avoid such occasional lapses is to recommit ourselves, each and every morning, to wellness, and to follow through that day with *whatever* actions are available to attain it.

THOUGHT FOR TODAY

One day at a time, I will do everything possible to ease the pain and heal the illness.

> "The worst pain a man can suffer: to have insight
> into much and power over nothing."
>
> HERODOTUS

If we are fortunate, serious illness and pain can bring about profound positive changes in our attitude and outlook. We can gain a more accurate perspective of our life in relation to the world around us, as well as a clear sense of what is important and what is not. These awarenesses enable us to forge rewarding new relationships with others, with God, and with ourselves.

By learning to live with uncertainty, we become more patient and more accepting. By fully realizing the futility and destructiveness of resentments, we become emotionally free, perhaps for the first time in our lives. By developing the ability to live in the moment, and to control our mind rather than letting it control us, we gain inner peace.

The greater challenge is to carry these awarenesses and lessons beyond illness and into the "outside world." When we are in remission, out of pain, or on the road to recovery, the goal is to *continue* practicing the principles we have learned.

Can we remain patient and accepting? Can we continue to forgive others and ourselves? Can we let go of pettiness and focus on what really matters? Can we move ever closer to God?

THOUGHT FOR TODAY
_____

What I learn from illness I will apply
to my larger life.

"Look not mournfully into the Past. It comes not back again. Wisely improve the present. It is time."

HENRY WADSWORTH LONGFELLOW

I never thought that chronic physical pain could be easier to endure than emotional pain. However, the truth is that few pains have been more agonizing and damaging than those I've caused myself by continuing to resent someone or something, by stubbornly refusing to forgive, and by self-destructively journeying back to the past.

When I dwell on painful memories I am certain to re-experience past suffering. When I rehash wrongs committed against me, I sentence myself to yet another term of bitterness and anguish. When I replay mistakes I have made and behavior I have regretted, I travel a road rutted with shame and guilt that leads nowhere.

Today I choose to travel in a new direction. I turn away from the past and return to the here and now. Today I will release the past and devote all my attention to the present. Today I will discard the pain-producing old ideas of yesterday. By doing so, I will again open myself to all the healing power, harmony, and serenity that God has to offer.

THOUGHT FOR TODAY

I will release the past, not relive it.

May 17

> "Self-confidence is the first requisite
> to great undertakings."
>
> SAMUEL JOHNSON

Many of us tend to focus more on our failures than our successes. In a typical scenario, we try to do something we've done dozens or even hundreds of times before: We swing a golf club, climb a flight of stairs, or make love. If we fail or only partially succeed, for one illness-related reason or another, our embarrassment is often compounded by feelings of disappointment and fear.

Then, the next time we want to begin one of those activities, a little voice inside our head insists that *we can't*. So we back off. Our plummeting self-confidence has become more of a disability than our actual physical limitations.

If our world is becoming smaller and smaller as the result of this cycle of negativity, we ought to remind ourselves that rebuilding self-confidence during illness is as important as rebuilding physical strength, emotional health, and spiritual connectedness. And we ought to pay close attention to every bit of progress, and make note of each of our successes.

THOUGHT FOR TODAY

Is my self-confidence crumbling?
Is it time for rebuilding?

"I shall light a candle of understanding in your heart,
which shall not be put out."

APOCRYPHA, II ESDRAS 14:25

A few weeks ago your wife suddenly started behaving as if your illness didn't exist. She stopped asking how you felt or if you needed anything. She stopped noticing that you were in pain, or depressed, or having trouble with your mobility.

Your first reaction was to leave her alone. You reasoned, "She's probably sick of me being sick. Who can blame her?" But after another week, her obliviousness to your condition began to seem not only strangely unlike her, but unkind. So you suggested a long-overdue heart-to-heart talk.

It took a while for both of you to realize what was going on. Quite a few tears were shed before the truth came out.

Your wife had become so frightened of your illness and its progression, and so frustrated with her inability to change its course in any way, that she "disassociated" herself. Quite unconsciously, she concluded that since she couldn't do anything to help, she might as well try to live her life as if nothing was wrong.

She had never stopped caring; you knew that all along. What you didn't fully realize was the depth of her frustration and sense of helplessness, and her need for greater understanding from you.

THOUGHT FOR TODAY

For everyone's sake, talk about it sooner, not later.

May 19

> "Fear, the very worst prophet in misfortune,
> anticipates many evils."
>
> STATIUS

The bills pour in and the paperwork accumulates: medical claims paid or rejected; overdue notices; hospital statements that are incomprehensible; and collection agency warnings that are all too clear.

We've tried to face the reality of assets minus liabilities, and coverage minus deductibles, as well as the prospect of having to borrow from relatives or file for bankruptcy. Yet in a sense, all of our financial footwork is beside the point. What is most overwhelming, and the one issue we haven't been able to deal with, is the tormenting *fear* of financial insecurity.

There is no better time than now to come to grips with that fear. Once we acknowledge that our negative projections are self-destructive scenarios that may never come to pass, we must do everything possible to live in the now, and deal only with today's actualities.

Since that is easier said than done, we can also ask for God's help. Many of us have learned that faith is the best antidote for fear. If we trust that God will provide for us, and if we *act* in faith by continuing to do today's footwork, our fears of future calamity are bound to diminish.

THOUGHT FOR TODAY

Fear of the future distorts the reality of the present.

"When water covers the head,
a hundred fathoms are as one."

PERSIAN PROVERB

Just before Easter last year it dawned on me that I was depressed and had been for several months. All that time I thought I was just tired, or possibly having some sort of biochemical reaction to chronic pain.

The more I thought about it, the more clearly I saw how my state of mind had been adversely affecting my life. Certainly the depression had dampened my enthusiasm for the physical activities—walking, gardening, even movie-going—that I normally enjoyed in spite of my illnesses. More seriously, the depression had somehow convinced me that my well-established regimen of meditation, exercise, and healthful diet choices was a waste of time. I had also been avoiding my friends, and because of my gloomy disposition, some of my friends and family members had been avoiding me.

Those of us who are chronically ill know full well that a certain amount of depression is par for the course. Indeed, depression is a necessary step in the process of grieving that leads to acceptance and peace of mind. However, when depression lingers and we are not able to move forward, it is time for action and assistance.

THOUGHT FOR TODAY

Is my state of mind leading me astray?

"Before you begin, get good counsel;
then, having decided, act promptly."

SALLUST

Depression during chronic illness may be inescapable, but it need not be inescapably permanent. There are a number of steps we can take to overcome depression and its effects.

An essential first step is to openly and honestly discuss the feelings of depression with your doctor. The condition could be a symptom of your illness, an illness in its own right, or the result of side effects or cross-reactions from medications. In any case, your doctor should be able to determine whether the depression can be overcome with relative ease, or is a condition requiring further medical treatment.

One of the best ways to overcome depression is to talk about it in a support group. By opening up about your feelings you will surely find that they are not uncommon, that you are hardly alone, and that you most certainly are not "losing your mind."

Many people believe that mild depression is a spiritual malady. In my own case I've learned that when I'm depressed I have almost always become "disconnected" from my own inner spirit. At that point I ask for God's help; I surrender and allow myself to be transformed and rejuvenated by His power and grace.

THOUGHT FOR TODAY

I may not feel like taking action, but
action can change my feelings.

"God helps everyone with
what is his own."

MIGUEL DE CERVANTES SAAVEDRA

Decisions, decisions. We thought there were quite enough to make in the old days: what classes to take, where to go on vacation, what movie to see, what to buy, what to wear. But those decisions were as nothing compared to the truly life-affecting ones we have to make these days.

Should we tell everyone about the illness, or just close friends and relatives? Should we try to go on working? Should we agree to an experimental treatment? Should we buy a wig now, or wait and see if the hair loss continues? Should we think about funeral arrangements? Are the kids too young to know?

Even when we get advice from friends or professionals, we don't always know if our decisions are the right ones. How can we be sure, when everything is so uncertain, and our life is changing so rapidly?

What assures and comforts us is knowing, deep down, that God's wisdom is always available. We turn to God in prayer and meditation, and before long we are again able to think clearly, choose confidently, and act decisively. God's love and gentle guidance leads us in the direction that is right for us, now and forever.

THOUGHT FOR TODAY

I can better decide with God at my side.

> "One must learn to love oneself with a wholesome
> and healthy love, so that one can bear to be
> with oneself and need not roam."
>
> FRIEDRICH NIETZSCHE

It's not uncommon for chronically ill people to lose their identity in the condition. Whoever we were prior to the onset of illness or injury—that is to say, the way we saw ourselves—can easily become overshadowed or replaced entirely by a new self-image based on suffering.

One reason is that people tend to treat us differently now that we are ill and in pain. They are solicitous and accommodating; they do their best to shield us from stress and even from reality, and they frequently watch their words in our presence. We are grateful for their concern and support, but we can't allow ourselves to be pushed ever deeper into the image of "illness sufferer."

Yes, the illness has brought about changes in our lifestyle; perhaps it's impossible, for now, to participate in certain activities that helped shape our identity. That doesn't mean the illness has to become our new identity.

Just because an illness takes up a great deal of our time and energy, we need not let it take over our entire being. We have the illness, we are not the illness. The illness is a part of us, not all of us.

THOUGHT FOR TODAY

I am a whole person, as before, facing
illness as one of life's challenges.

> "A man is not a wall, whose stones are crushed upon the road; or a pipe, whose fragments are thrown away at a street corner. The fragments of an intellect are always good."
>
> GEORGE SAND

At the hospital, and later at home, the feelings came flooding in. Some of them—like anxiety, confusion, anger—were relatively familiar. But other emotions were quite new to us. Never before had we experienced such depths of loneliness and despair. Even the familiar emotions were shockingly intense.

For a while these tumultuous feelings were almost as disturbing as the initial diagnosis, the treatment options, and the vague prognosis. During many long days and nights, we wondered which of our painful feelings were normal, which were irrational or abnormal, and how we would ever find our way through the shadowy maze.

Hesitantly at first, and then more forthrightly, we talked to our visitors—friends, relatives, nurses, other patients, counselors, clergy. And we were reassured that there is no "right" or "normal" way to feel. We came to understand that every one of our feelings reflects our individuality and represents, perhaps, a necessary stage in the recovery process.

We discovered that we could gain awareness from our feelings, change because of them, grow through them, or simply let them fade away without reacting at all.

THOUGHT FOR TODAY

There's no "right" way to feel.

May 25

> "For he that is used to go forward,
> and findeth a stop, falleth out of his own favour,
> and is not the thing he was."
>
> FRANCIS BACON

Nobody I know would ever expect of me what I demand of myself. Nobody I know would judge me so harshly. The problem is: I tend to judge myself during illness by the same stringent standards I applied when I was healthy.

This is not to say that *any* degree of self-judgment is in my best interest. However, the fact remains that sickness is (in addition to all else) a series of largely unavoidable personal embarrassments, disappointments, and failures. I overlook anniversaries and other important dates, miss deadlines, fall behind on bills, and lose patience with my loved ones. Almost daily I seem to fail at one thing or another, and then I feel that I've let everyone down.

God knows I would do things differently—*better*—if I could. But it's hard to improve performance when pain and fatigue erode my concentration and coordination.

So what can I do about it? I can try to lower my expectations, tailoring them to the realities of each new day. And, no matter how clumsy, forgetful, or frustrated I become, I can work and pray for acceptance—acceptance of myself exactly as I am right now.

THOUGHT FOR TODAY

The best I can do is good enough.

"Happiness is the only good. The time to be happy
is now. The place to be happy is here. The way
to be happy is to make others so."
ROBERT INGERSOLL

In those first discouraging days following the diagnosis of our illness, we were sure that life as we had known and enjoyed it was over. We felt that we would never again know happiness.

Soon we met others with the same illness. Many of them were happy, even joyous. Obviously they knew something we didn't. Or was it that they knew something we had forgotten?

The fact is that illness doesn't change a single basic truth about happiness. As our new friends reminded us, happiness is not an all-the-time thing or a forever thing, but a moment-to-moment thing. And it's up to us to recognize and savor each of those moments. They further reminded us that happiness doesn't come from the outside, but in all respects is an inside job.

Time has passed and we have learned a great deal more about the illness and ourselves. We can now affirm, from new experience, that happiness is not contingent on the state of our health, the state of our finances, or the attitudes and actions of others. We alone are responsible for it.

THOUGHT FOR TODAY

With illness now a part of my life, have I chosen not to
be happy? If so, am I willing to reverse that decision?

"Naught venture naught have."

JOHN HEYWOOD

You are not an especially passive person, but on the other hand you've always hated to "make waves." Now your disability has made it necessary to ask for special considerations at work. You have to tell your employer that you need to leave the office several times a week for physical therapy; you also need lower file cabinets and an office on the ground floor. And you dread the confrontation.

It's interesting, isn't it, that you see the need to be assertive as somehow "confrontational." It doesn't really have to be that way. While it's true that assertiveness can create stress, there are guidelines that can help you stay centered and self-confident.

First, remind yourself that you have the right motive for requesting changes. It's not that you are flexing your muscles, or trying to get something for nothing. Rather, your goal is to increase your capabilities in order to do a better job.

Second, it's probably a good idea to mentally rehearse the meeting with your boss. That way, you'll know exactly what to say and how to say it.

Finally, keep your priorities in order; remember that your health comes first. That's the whole purpose of your assertiveness.

THOUGHT FOR TODAY

Self-assertion need not be stressful.

"Life is a pure flame, and we live by
an invisible sun within us."

SIR THOMAS BROWNE

We've all had the experience of doing something thoughtful, caring, and perhaps unexpected for a friend or loved one, and then being surprised with an outpouring of heartfelt and gracious appreciation. When that happens we want to be even more thoughtful, more attentive, more kindly and considerate to that person.

Isn't that what life is like? When we are deeply thankful for each new day—when we have an attitude of gratitude for even simple pleasures—isn't it true that we continue to receive blessings, often unexpectedly?

Isn't that also what our spiritual connection is like? When we express heartfelt thanks to God we somehow broaden the channel of good and increase our capacity to recognize and receive His gifts.

We each have our own ways of expressing gratitude to God. We kneel and pray; we turn inward and simply say, "Thank you"; we speak through our actions by giving freely of ourselves to others.

Today and each day we give thanks to God for His presence in our lives. We are grateful for His love and guidance not only during times of great challenge, but also times of joy and tranquility.

THOUGHT FOR TODAY
_____

Am I open to goodness, to God's gifts,
to daily blessings?

> "We are but the instrument of Heaven.
> Our work is not design, but destiny."
>
> OWEN MEREDITH

A neighbor of mine is a surfer and professional yacht racer. One day, while talking with him about the beauty and power of the ocean, I described a near-death swimming experience I'd had some years earlier. I wondered aloud if he himself had ever feared an untimely "watery grave."

"I have a theory about that," he said. "If it's not your time to go, it's not going to happen. There have been too many times when I should have drowned and didn't."

I realized then that I feel very much as he does. I, too, have cheated death on more than a few occasions, surviving serious car wrecks and severed arteries; a coma resulting from a suicide attempt; malignant melanoma; and two heart attacks. People who know my history are amazed that I'm still alive.

But I'm not at all amazed. Those brushes with death, coupled with an ever-deeper trust that a loving God is in charge of my destiny, has convinced me that I'm alive today because that is His will. I believe, moreover, that He would have me do everything in my power to preserve, cherish, and fully savor this precious gift of life.

THOUGHT FOR TODAY

In God's time, according to God's plan, and with God's love.

"Action is eloquence."

WILLIAM SHAKESPEARE

You've been home from the hospital for two months and depression has given way to boredom. There's never anything on TV, or so it seems. One night, in desperation, you began to count the flowers on the living-room wallpaper. Following that, you blurted out to your partner, "We never go anywhere, we never do anything. We never have fun any more!"

We've all had outbursts like that. We forget that "fun activities" don't just happen by themselves even when we're in the best of health. They usually have to be discussed, planned, and scheduled. They have to flow from an enthusiastic desire rather than a sense of self-pity.

Moreover, when we are ill it's easy to become overly protective of ourselves, to "cocoon." It's tempting to let negative emotions drag us down and convince us (with irony we're unaware of) that having fun isn't worth the effort.

If some of this sounds familiar, perhaps it's time to reorder your priorities, to do some research and find out what activities you can enjoy within your new limitations. There's no better time than now to start having fun again.

THOUGHT FOR TODAY

Just because I can't be a social butterfly, that doesn't mean I have to remain in my cocoon.

May 31

"Human beings, by changing the inner attitudes of their minds, can change the outer aspects of their lives."

WILLIAM JAMES

We've never disputed the idea that so long as we are alive we have choices. However, considering the fact that our physical capabilities have diminished, severely so for some of us, it's sometimes difficult to recognize what choices are left.

Even if we do face physical limitations, we continue to have an abundance of mental, emotional, and attitudinal choices. We can choose to pursue inner peace by living a day at a time; by working to overcome self-centeredness; and by practicing spiritual principles.

We can choose hope by opening ourselves to the positive experiences of others; by refusing to indulge in self-pitying and despairing thoughts; by taking a leadership role in our health care; and by trusting God.

We can choose love and connectedness by saying no to judgmentalism and cynicism, and by reaching out appreciatively and empathetically to friends, family members, and others who are ill.

THOUGHT FOR TODAY

Positive choices have the potential
to move me toward wellness.

June

June 1

"I don't use drugs.
My dreams are frightening enough."

MARIE E. ESCHENBACH

I never thought I'd envy people who have serious yet curable illnesses, but sometimes I do. For them, pain strikes and then leaves, fever rises but soon drops. They are sick, but they know they will get well. Chronic illness makes none of those promises. The road is occasionally smooth and level, often rutted and steep, and always unpredictable. We never really know what's around the next curve.

In my own case, one of the "unpredictables" is the way my mind twists and turns when I'm at my worst, bedridden and in pain. I sometimes experience recurring daydreams and nightmares that seem frighteningly real.

God comes to visit and His disapproval of me is clearly evident. Of course, I am being punished, deservedly so, and this is only the beginning . . .

I am dying, and everything I have come to believe about the transition and the journey is untrue. There is no light, no warmth, and no familiar faces.

Thankfully, the ghastly images never stay with me. When I awaken or return to the here and now, I accept them for the biochemical distortions that they are. I let them flow by with neither claim nor regret.

THOUGHT FOR TODAY

Only reality is real.

"What annoyances are more painful than those
of which we cannot complain?"
MARQUIS DE CUSTINE

At a lupus support-group meeting recently, we talked about our tendency to automatically respond "fine" when people ask us how we are feeling, even when we're hurting. We concluded that it was time for each of us to be more forthright when answering questions about our health.

A week later the group leader phoned to chat. "How are you feeling?" she asked me. "Fine," I responded reflexively. Actually, I was in the middle of a painful flare-up. After a brief pause, we both laughed.

Why are we so often reluctant to let others know how we are really feeling? For one thing, we may fear being labeled complainers or hypochondriacs. For another, we may think people are asking about our health just to be polite. Perhaps, too, we don't want to burden others with the responsibility of comforting us. Or, we may still be in denial, unwilling to admit to ourselves (let alone anyone else) how we're actually feeling.

These are all possible motives for saying "fine" when we're not. In any case, the next time someone asks how we're doing, let's at least think about it briefly before automatically responding in the usual way.

THOUGHT FOR TODAY
How am I feeling? Am I really "fine"?

June 3

> "'He means well' is useless
> unless he does well."
>
> PLAUTUS

On your nightstand next to the phone there's a carefully prepared list of all the things you can do to hasten healing. And you're going to work your way through that list. You are going to start keeping a medical journal, attending a support group, and exercising regularly. You are going to start reading all those pamphlets and books you've collected, and really educate yourself about the illness. And you are definitely going to find ways to eliminate toxic stress from your life— but not this week.

First, you have to find someone to take over the gardening chores and someone to carpool the kids; there are two months' worth of bills to be paid and recorded; the car needs a tune-up; and there's also the…. Wait a minute. What's going on here? Is it possible that your priorities are slightly awry?

Getting well has to come first. It has to take precedence over *all else* in your life—not simply household chores and financial matters, but also community and social obligations, job responsibilities and even family relationships. Getting well is everything; there's nothing more important.

THOUGHT FOR TODAY
_____

First things first.

"All these woes shall serve,
For sweet discourses in our time to come."
WILLIAM SHAKESPEARE

One of the things that can make illness more acceptable, or at least more tolerable, is the expectation that we will come through it with a degree of spiritual enlightenment. Our suffering is tempered by the sense that we'll become more self-aware and capable as the result of our experiences, and that our life will be enriched.

Are these hopes realistic and achievable? Or, by such projection, are we simply trying to avoid the harsh actualities of chronic illness and pain?

Those of us who have "been there" can attest that illness does indeed offer boundless opportunities for personal and spiritual growth. We have found that when we approach sickness and healing creatively and imaginatively, in the spirit of self-discovery, we can greatly improve the quality of our inner life.

Illness certainly encourages us to adjust our perspective and reorder our priorities, so we are able to see clearly what is important and what is not. Moreover, illness offers us the opportunity to gain humility. By virtue of our suffering we become better able to understand others— to be empathetic, compassionate, and forgiving.

THOUGHT FOR TODAY

Illness can strengthen my spiritual beliefs and
bring me closer to my Higher Power.

June 5

When the doctor detailed the nature of our illness, hardly anyone could tell how overwhelmed with fear we actually were. It's amazing how creatively we disguised our true feelings, especially from ourselves.

For some of us, fear masqueraded as anger; we raged and railed at everything and everybody, from the FDA to nurses who had trouble inserting intravenous needles. Or we sublimated our fear by indulging in self-pity, by criticizing anyone who crossed us, and by finding fault with every aspect of our treatment. In short, we managed to avoid the real issue—the illness and our actual feelings about it—by focusing on things outside of us.

Our avoidance made things a lot tougher for everyone than they had to be. We created tremendous stress, wasted valuable energy, and antagonized the healthcare professionals who were doing their very best to treat us.

Looking back, it's quite clear how we detoured ourselves from the path of recovery and wellness during those early days. And the lessons we learned—especially the need to deal honestly with our feelings as they arise—serve us well to this day.

THOUGHT FOR TODAY

Am I still attempting to disguise "unacceptable" emotions?

"There is no truth.
There is only perception."
GUSTAVE FLAUBERT

My dog was once sideswiped by a car when he raced across the street. It took months for him to recover. Watching him play the other day, I realized that even though he's been back to his old self for quite some time, I still think of him as fragile.

That awareness helped me better understand why certain friends and relatives treat me with kid gloves. They continue to see me as delicate and vulnerable, as if I'm always on the verge of collapse. They still treat me carefully and speak in grave tones when they ask about my health. When they focus all that attention on my illness to the exclusion of just about everything else in my life, I become uncomfortable and sometimes even angry.

I realize now that they are not the problem, and that it's up to me to overcome my feelings of discomfort. I can tell them that I appreciate their ongoing concern, but that I'm now ready for the relationship to return to "normal." I can also try to be more understanding of them, and not let their words and actions influence my improving self-image.

THOUGHT FOR TODAY

Do I still see myself as somewhat fragile and perhaps present myself to others that way?

June 7

> "He who fears he shall suffer,
> already suffers what he fears."
>
> MICHEL EYQUEM DE MONTAIGNE

When we were very young, four or five years old, a scraped knee or elbow was cause for inconsolable sobbing, with the expectation of much sympathy and attention from our parents. In our teenage years, such behavior was "uncool"; pain wasn't supposed to faze us, and for the most part it didn't.

The point, of course, is that the way we feel and behave when pain strikes has as much to do with our reaction as it does to the actual pain itself. While this may seem fairly obvious, it is a vital reality, one that we should try to keep at the forefront of our consciousness when we are experiencing chronic pain.

This is not to say that we should pretend our pain doesn't exist, or that we should refuse to treat it with all the means available to us. Rather, we need to become ever more aware of our attitudes about pain, and our reactions to it. While we may not be able to make the pain disappear entirely, we certainly can reduce the suffering it causes us by changing our expectations of it.

THOUGHT FOR TODAY

I may be powerless over the pain, but I do
have power over my reactions to it.

> "A man's own observation, what he finds
> good of and what he finds hurt of, is the
> best physic to preserve health."
>
> FRANCIS BACON

When I unexpectedly saw my refection in a shop window I was taken aback. Hunched over, chin tilted downward, I appeared shorter, smaller, and sort of gathered in. I hardly recognized myself.

After thinking dejectedly about the experience and then, several days later, discussing it with my rheumatologist, I realized what had been taking place. My posture was being seriously affected, first of all, by the disease process itself—inflammation, stiffness, and pain. Because of these symptoms, I was frequently exhausted and depressed. And the more I was pulled down physically and emotionally, the less I felt like holding myself upright. Years of low self-esteem also contributed to my poor posture, I'm quite sure of that.

It is well documented that rounded shoulders and a slumping stance can cause or increase back pain, muscle tension, and headaches. Poor posture can also diminish breathing capability and interfere with digestion. On the bright side, improvement in posture often leads to improvement in physical movement and capability. With proper posture, moreover, energy and vitality increase, while muscular tension and pain levels decrease.

THOUGHT FOR TODAY

Is poor posture part of the reason
I'm feeling poorly?

> "Nothing is so easy but it becomes difficult
> when done with reluctance."
>
> TERENCE

Illness robs us of so much control and choice that we want to sound the trumpets when we discover an area of life where we can regain some control. One such area is posture, which, as we're learning, can affect our state of mind, self-image, and physical health either adversely or beneficially.

Of course, it's one thing to see the potential but quite another to follow through with actions that can turn potential into actuality. Bearing that in mind, here are some suggested techniques for developing and maintaining good posture.

The first step is to become constantly aware of the position and alignment of your body. How are you sitting right now, for example, as you are reading this page? Check and correct your posture many times each day. If you do that conscientiously, good posture will eventually become second nature.

"Think tall" at all times, not only when you are standing and walking, but also when you are sitting or lying down.

Periodically, check your posture by looking at your reflection in a mirror or store window, or by standing with your back against a wall. Your partner can help with gentle reminders.

THOUGHT FOR TODAY

Think tall.

"Our remedies oft in ourselves do lie,
which we ascribe to heaven."
WILLIAM SHAKESPEARE

There is a lot more to health care and healing than keeping doctors' appointments and taking pills. For many of us the journey to wellness is as much an inner spiritual one as it is a medical one. We strongly believe that our attitudes, emotions, and actions have a profound influence on our physical health.

That is why we try to live life a day at a time, making the most of each moment as it unfolds. We avoid fearful projection into the future, as well as guilt-burdened excursions into the past.

The way we see it, there's no better time than now to deal with unresolved issues that can divert our energy from healing. We do our best to recognize and release our resentments, to make amends for hurtful behavior, and to truly forgive those who have harmed us. Instead of automatically focusing on what we perceive as bad or wrong in life, we look for the good in others and in the world around us.

Through prayer and meditation we seek and strive to do God's will: to be of service; to share our experience, strength, and hope; to let love flow freely.

THOUGHT FOR TODAY

Harness your inner resources.

June 11

"Sorrow makes us all children again."

RALPH WALDO EMERSON

Through a good part of the treatment process, including surgery, we were cushioned and numbed by denial. Time passed; denial gradually evolved into anger, then depression, and finally acceptance.

Here we are, months later, and denial is back. This time, however, it belongs to certain friends and family members who are unwilling or unable to face the seriousness of our condition. They find the possibility of our death so hard to bear that they have convinced themselves we're doing quite well.

Such reactions are understandable, but they are terribly hard on us. It takes an enormous amount of energy to go along with the pretense that everything is just wonderful. The burden of sustaining someone else's fiction can force us to withdraw, which increases our sense of loneliness.

It's extremely difficult to deal with denial of this sort. We have to weigh the fragility of our loved ones' emotional states against the effect of their denial on us, before deciding what to do. Whenever possible, it's probably best to try to bring them around to reality. In some cases, unfortunately, an understanding of their behavior may be as far as we're able to go.

THOUGHT FOR TODAY

I pray that my loved ones will find acceptance.

"Let nothing disturb you, let nothing frighten you,
All things pass away. God never changes.
Patience obtains all things. He who has God finds
he lacks nothing. God alone suffices."

ST. TERESA OF AVILA

The cardiologist drew a little diagram of my coronary arteries. He showed me how the blockages had been surgically bypassed with four new grafts. Then he said, not unkindly, "Now the rest is up to you. Low-fat diet, exercise, maintain your weight, and avoid stress."

No problem, I quickly concluded. My weight was okay, I swam regularly, and I was quite willing to give up eggs, hot dogs, and junk food.

As for stress, I didn't really think there was any in my life. Yet in reality I was experiencing all sorts of stress-inducing events and attitudes. I just hadn't been able to recognize them and the effects they were having on me.

What turned me around was a simple yet powerful suggestion from a rehab nurse. She recommended that I write out a stress inventory each day, detailing specific events and my mental, physical, and emotional reactions to them.

What happened when I got stuck in traffic? What did I do when an insurance payment to me was late? How did I react to pain, to fear, to a seeming lack of understanding by someone close? Little did I know, and how much I have learned!

THOUGHT FOR TODAY

Stress detours me away from wellness.

> "All is change;
> all yields its place and goes."
>
> EURIPIDES

There will be days—perhaps this is such a one—when you will feel awful. Awfully sick, awfully alone, awfully angry. You won't want to be encouraged by one more person—neither mother, nor father, nor loving partner, nor kindly doctor. You won't be able to accept comfort from friends, inspiration from readings, or strength from God. You will be inconsolable.

You will wonder, "Has it always been like this? Will I always feel this way? Won't it ever change?"

Pursue that last thought and hold fast to it. The inevitability of change will be your thread of hope, the directional marker that can bring you to a different state of mind and a more realistic frame of reference.

You will begin to remember that, *no*, you haven't always felt this way, and that *yes*, it will change for the better. You will become willing again to accept comfort. Your faith will be rekindled and you will turn once more to God for courage and strength.

Painful days may well come your way from time to time. When they do, hang on the best way you can until they pass, for they surely will.

THOUGHT FOR TODAY

I will focus on the inevitability
of change.

"Death is but crossing the world, as friends do the seas;
they live in one another still."

WILLIAM PENN

The two of you are as close as a couple can be. You've been through some really tough times together and the relationship has grown stronger with each experience. Neither of you could ever have dreamed being as intimate, on so many levels, with another person; there's nothing you haven't talked about or explored together.

Except for one thing; you haven't yet talked about death, and the time to do so may be growing short.

You each have your reasons for avoiding the subject. As the caregiver, you have felt that any mention of death or dying would bring you to tears, and you can't imagine anything more upsetting to your partner. As the one who is ill, you have tiptoed around the subject for the same reason, plus one other: You don't want your partner to feel you've given up hope.

Clearly, this is the time to step out of the shadows, to let the love you have for each other work even greater magic. This is the time to share your beliefs, ideas, fears, and past experiences regarding death. This is the time to give the very best of yourself—strength, comfort, and reassurance.

THOUGHT FOR TODAY

The "right moment" is the one
you choose or create.

June 15

> "Therefore keep in the midst of life. Do not isolate yourself. Be among men and things, and among troubles, and difficulties, and obstacles."
>
> HENRY DRUMMOND

Sometimes, because we've had several bad days in a row (or for no apparent reason at all), we cross an invisible line. It separates patience from exasperation, tolerance from irritability, acceptance from defiance, and hope from despair. Once on the other side of that line, we become easily annoyed by almost everything and everybody.

The oatmeal tastes different. The wind is too loud. The pillow smells funny. And there are too many people around.

When we reach that point, all we want to do is insulate and isolate ourselves from the rest of the world. So we unplug the phone, turn off the lights, pull down the shade, and pull up the covers. It seems that we have no other choice.

But of course most of the time we do have a choice, one that is very important to recognize. While it can be beneficial to go off by ourselves occasionally, it's never in our interest to shut out the larger world, to shun human contact for any substantial length of time, and to deprive ourselves of the love and caring that is available to us in such abundance.

THOUGHT FOR TODAY

I'm not always in the best possible company when I'm alone.

"If time be of all things the most precious,
wasting time must be the greatest prodigality."
BENJAMIN FRANKLIN

Today has the potential to be very special. It is bright and brand-new, unlike any other day in the past or yet to come. Today is a priceless and precious gift to me from God, and I will try to live it gratefully and joyously.

It is my desire and intention to experience this day—physically, emotionally, and spiritually—to the fullest extent of my capabilities. I will try not to let the hours drag by, slip by, or pass unnoticed. Rather, I will savor each one as it unfolds, and make the most of it within the present circumstances of my life.

On this very special day, I give God my full attention. I will focus on His unconditional love for me and my fellows. I will try to think and act in ways that bear witness to that immutable reality.

I affirm that I will live this new day in the spirit of harmony, tranquility, gratitude, and service. In all my involvements with friends, family members, and acquaintances, I will strive to be an instrument of God's grace.

THOUGHT FOR TODAY

How can I best live this precious
new day?

June 17

"Criticism should not be querulous and wasting,
all knife and root-puller, but guiding, instructive,
inspiring, a south wind, not an east wind."

RALPH WALDO EMERSON

The decision to criticize someone is always a tough call, all the more so when the person on the receiving end is a healthcare professional or a caregiver. It's hard to be critical of doctors, nurses, and supportive family members who, for the most part, have been helpful, caring, and dependable. Rather than appear ungrateful, we may be tempted to "look the other way," and there certainly are times when that's the right thing to do.

We should carefully and objectively weigh the importance of the issue at hand before we actually criticize someone. It's wise to choose our battles, so to speak, when physical and emotional energy is at a premium. Moreover, we ought to be absolutely sure that our motive for criticism is constructive, and that we are not simply being self-righteous or trying to "get even."

Once we've decided that something definitely needs to be said, in the interest of long-term harmony we should try to make our point thoughtfully and gently. For example, we can offer helpful suggestions along with our criticism, and we can also sweeten our words with a compliment if that's appropriate.

THOUGHT FOR TODAY

Before I criticize I will carefully examine
my motives and weigh my words.

> "Friendship adds a brighter radiance to
> prosperity and lightens the burden of adversity
> by dividing and sharing it."
>
> CICERO

We will always be grateful to our close friends. They were right there when we needed them, when our illness was out of control and we had no idea where it would lead. They chauffeured us, fed us, took care of our kids, calmed our fears, brought us back to earth, and even made us laugh when nothing was really funny. They were blessings, those dear friends, and they still are.

Time has passed, and we've come to terms with the illness. It no longer completely dominates our thoughts, but has become an accepted part of life. We feel confident and emotionally strong again. We're eager to "move on," so to speak, and to give back some of what we've received.

It's important for us to tell our friends that we've become more independent and capable. We can ask them now to put aside their "helper" roles and rejoin us in the two-way friendship of earlier days. It will be such a pleasure to return to the shared thoughts, feelings, and interests that led to compatibility and closeness in the first place.

THOUGHT FOR TODAY

God's grace often comes
in the form of friends.

> "It's not what he has, nor even what he does, which
> directly expresses the worth of a man, but what he is."
>
> HENRI FRÉDÉRIC AMIEL

Many of us can see now that we derived much of our self-worth from our avocations and occupations. As athletes, for example, our identities flowed from the ability to run a marathon or power a mountain bike up a steep trail. As professionals, we measured our worth by productivity, creativity, and the financial rewards we received. Some of us also valued ourselves according to our physical appearance.

When illness roared into our lives, the foundations of our identities crumbled and our self-worth soon followed. We were devastated because we could barely swing a golf club or run once around the block. We were humiliated because we missed deadlines, lost time from work, and felt thoroughly incompetent. And we were mortified by the way we looked.

Those of us who have taken this kind of fall had been measuring our value on the wrong scales. We've since learned that true and lasting self-worth comes not from what we do for a living or for fun, but from who we are—from such valuable *inner* qualities as courage, kindness, honesty, faith, and humility. These are the qualities we continue to nurture, the ones that will thrive no matter what our physical condition.

THOUGHT FOR TODAY

Do I sometimes feel that illness has depreciated
my value as a person?

"Time deals gently only with those
who take it gently."

ANATOLE FRANCE

I once visited a clock museum in Furtwangen, Germany. The sprawling building was filled with timepieces of every size and description, from ancient sundials and liturgical masterpieces to ornately carved cuckoo clocks and Space Age wristwatches.

I reflected, as I wandered through the museum, that timekeeping is a hallmark of civilization, an indication of people's need and desire to organize and structure their lives productively. As my eyes began to glaze over with images of countless clocks, it further occurred to me that all too often we are tyrannized by time because of the way we perceive it.

Those of us who are ill, in particular, tend to develop a negative relationship with time, in the sense that it is "dragging" or being "wasted." Or we see time as an enemy, standing between us and relief from our pain.

Whenever I become trapped in such a relationship, through obsessive clock-watching or similar obsessions, I think back to that clock museum in the Black Forest. By visualizing shelves upon shelves and rooms upon rooms of *all those clocks* (the cuckoo clocks especially), I am able to recognize and smile at the absurdity of my behavior.

THOUGHT FOR TODAY

Am I tyrannized by time?

June 21

> "Better to ask a question
> than to remain ignorant."
>
> PROVERB

It's 3:30 a.m. and you are suddenly wide awake, bedeviled by a pack of nipping, nagging questions. This is the third night in a row you've lost sleep, fearfully wondering what the doctor meant. Being ill would probably be easier to bear if there weren't so many *unknowns*.

The doctor said you wouldn't be able to walk for a while. *Does that mean a week, a month, or what?* The nurse told you to call if you have any side effects. *What side effects—nausea, dizziness, sleeplessness?* The counselor said you have to learn to accept the illness. *How do I do that? What does that involve?*

While it's true that some health questions can't be answered definitively, if at all, many questions can be answered with precision and clarity. The problem is not that the information is unavailable, but that we as patients or caregivers hesitate to take charge of the question-and-answer process. All too often we are intimidated or embarrassed to ask for elaboration or clarification.

We shouldn't have to assume or wonder about anything. So let's ask the doctor. Let's ask the nurse. Let's ask someone else with the same illness. Let's ask, and if necessary ask again and again.

THOUGHT FOR TODAY

The answer may not be readily available,
but I won't know unless I ask.

"It is hidden wrath that harms."

SENECA

Anyone who has ever been seriously injured and forced to live with unrelenting pain is familiar with the special kind of anger that rises out of these conditions. We are angry that we have been "singled out" and that we have lost control over so many aspects of our lives.

Some of us vent our rage in the form of antagonism and spitefulness toward those around us. Others suppress this volatile emotion, perhaps hoping it will somehow dissipate.

Anger dealt with in either of these ways can have as much of a negative effect on our lives as the disabling conditions that caused it in the first place. We're all familiar with the strained relationships, guilt, headaches, backaches, and sleeplessness that result from anger suppressed or denied.

How can we deal with this normal and even necessary emotion? One of the best ways is to talk about our anger, perhaps trying to describe it, thereby making some sense of it. For example, when we realize there is no real justification for our anger that alone may lessen its power. Verbalizing anger, especially to someone in the same boat, can go a long way toward alleviating it.

THOUGHT FOR TODAY

In order to accept my illness, I must first come to terms with my anger about it.

June 23

> "These are thy glorious works,
> Parent of good."
>
> JOHN MILTON

We know how illness can trigger massive distortions in our ability to see things right-size while clouding our ability to perceive things as they really are. All too frequently when we are in the grip of illness, we focus wholly on the seemingly negative limitations of our lives, while overlooking the blessings that continue to flow into and around us.

The reality is that each of us has a Divine heritage. God's eternal will for us, in sickness or in health, is good and only good. None of the challenges we face—neither pain, nor natural disaster, nor financial hardship, nor hostility from others—can prevent us from receiving God's gifts of strength, guidance, love, and spiritual abundance.

In order to fully avail ourselves of these precious gifts, we are learning to more willingly let go and let God. We try to do so not only when we are clearly powerless, but on a regular basis. When we let go of *all* our concerns and let God's will prevail, it is then that we regain a clear view and true perspective. We are comforted; we are tranquil; we are grateful.

THOUGHT FOR TODAY

I acknowledge my Divine heritage. I will open
my mind and heart to God's grace.

> "Friends, if we be honest with ourselves, we shall
> be honest with each other."
>
> GEORGE MACDONALD

Last summer one of my daughters traveled cross-country to visit. Even though I was suffering through a major lupus flare-up, we were able to have a great week together.

The night before my daughter's early morning flight back home, I stubbornly insisted on driving her to the airport, despite the fact that it would mean getting up at 5:00 a.m. Both my daughter and wife tried to talk me out of it; they pointed out that it would take me days to recover from a night of insufficient rest. All evening I refused to listen to reason. Finally, at bedtime, I conceded and agreed to let my wife drive to the airport.

When I awakened the next morning at 10:00 a.m., still tired and in considerable pain even after a full night's sleep, I realized that I hadn't played fair with my family. I had pridefully tried to ignore a major reality in all of our lives and, in the process, had caused unnecessary stress for everyone.

Hopefully the lesson will stay with me. Playing fair means realistically evaluating the state of my illness and its expected course, and then, honestly communicating that information.

THOUGHT FOR TODAY

Forthrightness and honesty build
acceptance and trust.

June 25

"We often pretend to fear what we really despise,
and more often despise what we really fear."

CHARLES CALEB COLTON

When people don't understand an illness and therefore fear it, they often stigmatize those who have it. AIDS is the most obvious example at present, but other illnesses, including cancer, muscular dystrophy, multiple sclerosis, and lupus are also stigmatized in varying degrees for the same reason.

What is it that people fear about our illnesses? They are afraid that the disease will somehow rub off on them and taint their lives. Out of ignorance and self-centeredness, they fear not only contagion but also their own emotional confusion.

When we are fighting a debilitating and life-threatening illness, we don't need the added burdens of negative judgments, ridicule, and shame. We don't need to torment ourselves worrying whether or not to disclose the illness.

Stigmatization is a serious problem that can cause tremendous stress. It is not an issue that should be left unresolved. To the contrary, it must be dealt with and worked through, with whatever resources are available, from family members and support groups to social-service workers and professional counselors.

THOUGHT FOR TODAY

Do I sometimes stigmatize myself?

"I will have no locked cupboards in my life."
GERTRUDE BELL

Stigmatization is poisonous and painful, but those of us who are its targets need not accept the heartache. We are not the problem; the real problems are misinformation, ignorance, and fear. Whether the illness in our lives is a blatantly stigmatized one such as TB or Addiction, or one where the stigma is more subtle, there are steps we can take to avoid or shed this unnecessary burden.

Before we move from silence to disclosure, we ought to decide carefully whom we want to tell. While it's generally not a good idea to remain secretive about any illness, that doesn't mean every single person in our lives has to be given a complete rundown.

In some cases, there are advantages in gradually releasing or "staging" information. That way, we can prepare others emotionally and soften the impact.

When we open up about an illness, we should remember that we are doing so primarily to reduce the emotional pressure on ourselves. One way to accomplish this is by educating others and letting them know what we are going through. Hopefully they will respond with compassion and kindness, and even offer a helping hand.

THOUGHT FOR TODAY

How can I best replace ignorance with information, and fear with understanding?

June 27

"Change, the strongest son of life."
GEORGE MEREDITH

The pain of my chronic joint inflammation changes from hour to hour and day to day. There is little I can do to control its onset or severity. When I first faced that reality, I was distraught and ready to give up on my body.

I constructed dismal scenarios of my future life. I would have to hire people—a gardener, a handyman—to do the things I had always enjoyed, or maybe someone to run errands. I'd have to stop riding my bike. I'd have to give up long walks with my wife as well as other physical activities, including sex.

As time passed and my despairing thoughts gradually dissipated, this is what I realized: For now I may be powerless over the joint inflammation, but I'm certainly not powerless over how I approach, deal with, and work around the chronic pain.

I start by doing everything possible to keep my body strong and flexible. Following that, I carefully approach the activities most likely to be restricted by my condition. Cautiously, patiently, and sometimes experimentally, I work within (and around) my physical limitations. So far I haven't had to give up anything entirely. I've simply had to learn to do things differently.

THOUGHT FOR TODAY

Do I give up too soon?

"Never hurry. Take plenty of exercise.
Always be cheerful. Take all the sleep you need.
You may expect to be well."

JAMES FREEMAN CLARKE

Few of us ever ran marathons or scaled rock faces, but we did enjoy more moderate forms of exercise. When illness came, we at first thought we would have to forgo our workouts, but we eventually discovered that for most of us exercise is not only possible but necessary.

Just about anyone can do some kind of exercise. Even if it has been months or years since you've exercised, and even if you are confined to a bed or wheelchair, starting up again can be as simple as finding the forms and techniques that are right for your condition.

Once you've gotten your doctor's input and approval, you can begin to establish a regular routine. Your primary guideline should be "easy does it." That is, don't set unrealistic goals and don't push yourself. Listen to the wisdom of your body and exercise until you feel good, not until you are wiped out.

You can look forward to a gradual increase in energy and self-esteem. You'll feel stronger, more flexible, and more capable. Your breathing will deepen, your color will brighten, and you will sleep more soundly. Best of all, you will take pride in the fact that you are helping yourself to get well again.

THOUGHT FOR TODAY

So long as I live and breathe, I will do all
in my power to grow stronger.

> "Solitude vivifies;
> isolation kills."
>
> JOSEPH ROUX

We're never quite sure how we will be feeling from one day to the next, so we hesitate to make plans or commitments. We feel somewhat ashamed of our illness, as if it's somehow a sign of personal weakness. Besides that, we don't want people to see us unless we look our best. And we certainly don't want to be around friends who will remind us of our former lifestyle, who will tell us how good the skiing has been, or how well things are going at work.

So we gradually shut ourselves off from the world, until we are completely isolated. We begin to live inside of our own mind, which is hardly the safest place to be. Before long every symptom, ache, pain, uncertainty, concern, and fear is magnified tenfold. We lose touch with reality. We also lose touch with hope, optimism, faith, and especially the healing power of love.

Thankfully, it doesn't take much to bring us back. A nice lunch with a close friend can do it. A walk through the neighborhood and a look upward at the trees and sky can help us realize what we've been missing. Once our spirit is revitalized, we begin to thrive again.

THOUGHT FOR TODAY

I choose God's larger world over the solitary confinement of my mind.

> "Next to the assumption of power was
> the responsibility of relinquishing it."
>
> BENJAMIN DISRAELI

We've been told repeatedly how important it is to retain as much control of our daily lives as possible. The reason, of course, is that chronic illness wrests so much control away from us. But in certain areas we may have to *relinquish* control.

Some of us are used to being in charge. We've run a household or a business, and people have depended on us. Now, however, it's time to be more flexible in our relationships, and to modify our "leadership" role. It's time to give ourselves permission to have a chronic illness, and to put our health needs above all else.

As parents, for example, it may be necessary to give our children more responsibilities; they may have to grow up more quickly than we would have wished. Similarly, it may be necessary to delegate some authority at work or in community activities.

After years or perhaps a lifetime of being "in charge," it may take a while to change our role and trust that others are capable of carrying on with less involvement on our part. In the long run, however, it's likely that everyone will benefit.

THOUGHT FOR TODAY

I am not indispensable.

July

> "We carry with us the wonders
> we seek without us."
>
> SIR THOMAS BROWNE

The feelings—disappointment, sadness, shame—sometimes come out of nowhere. Or they may be brought on by an actual occurrence or image, such as an awards ceremony, a sports event, an ebullient phone call from a friend on vacation. We thought we had finally grown used to our illness and gained acceptance, but once again we are dragged down by our regretful and bitter emotions.

We are disappointed because certain career and personal goals seem out of reach. We are sad because we can't charge through life the way we once did. And we are ashamed because just about everyone we know has passed us by and is getting more, doing more, being more.

Thank God we're learning how to confront these tormenting feelings. We're learning how to cry out "Stop!" when we begin comparing our life today to our life in the past; when we begin to yearn for the life we had hoped for; when we begin to envy the lives of others.

Self-acceptance is our goal. Each time we are able to achieve it, or move closer to it—each time we are able to catch ourselves and back away from those hurtful comparisons—we feel relieved and whole again.

THOUGHT FOR TODAY

Right now I'm everything
I'm meant to be.

July 2

> "To the sick, while there
> is life there is hope."
>
> CICERO

Not long ago, I had a really good week, the kind that can send my hopes and spirits soaring. When I responded to the rheumatologist's first question by saying, "Just fine," his eyes sparkled and he cracked a rare smile. And when my brother phoned that same week, I could hear the joy in his voice after I proudly announced that I'd been feeling great.

The next time around, when I wasn't doing well at all, I hesitated before replying truthfully to the expectant queries of doctors, family members, and friends. I felt somehow obligated to remain "in the pink" and on the upswing. I guess I didn't want to cause disappointment or sadness, or give anyone the impression that I was perhaps failing to take proper care of myself.

People with chronic illnesses are under tremendous pressure—from themselves as well as others—to get well quickly and return to their "normal, productive lives." However, we can't let these pressures build to the point where they distort reality and interfere with the acceptance of our illness. We'd rather not be sick, but we are, and we're learning to live with it the best way we can.

THOUGHT FOR TODAY

Share the hope, but
spare the pressure.

"But wonder on, till truth
makes all things plain."

WILLIAM SHAKESPEARE

Illness often strikes without warning. Following the initial shock, some of us may be troubled by a sense of personal failure. We feel ashamed for becoming ill, and even more ashamed that the illness has lingered. We hate to talk about our illness, because when we do, some people volunteer theories about the things we did to make ourselves sick, while others suggest steps we should be taking to get well. In either case, we feel ashamed for not "doing right."

Adding to our sense of personal failure is society's message that excellent health is the norm, and that anything deviating from such perfection is therefore abnormal. Of course, nothing could be further from the truth.

When we feel a sense of personal failure for becoming sick and staying sick, we're assuming that we have power over the advent, timing, and extent of our illnesses. Yet in fact we are utterly powerless in this area.

For some of us, this is a hard truth to swallow; we've been conditioned to believe otherwise. However, the sooner we are able to acknowledge, accept, and take spiritual advantage of our powerlessness, the sooner the painful notion of "personal failure" will become a mere memory.

THOUGHT FOR TODAY

Self-recrimination has no place
in the recovery process.

> "Freedom is the supreme good—
> freedom from self-imposed limitation."
>
> ELBERT HUBBARD

There will be fireworks tonight, picnics and parades. As I celebrate our nation's independence, I will also set aside a special time to celebrate my own personal freedom.

I once thought freedom meant being able to go anywhere and do anything, without restrictions of any kind. I have since come to believe that freedom is far more than the absence of physical limitations.

My mind holds the key to personal freedom. So long as I create limitations within myself, that is how long I will remain in bondage. So long as I am able to rise above self-created limitations that is how long I will enjoy freedom.

There may be times when I am unable to join others or easily move about, but I can rise above my external existence. I am a beloved child of God, and my spirit is forever free.

Thanks to God, I am learning to transcend illness and pain. Thanks to God, the shackles of despair are being replaced with the wings of hope. Thanks to God, I am free.

THOUGHT FOR TODAY

Now and always, I celebrate
freedom of the spirit.

"Life is not measured
by the time we live."
GEORGE CRABBE

There has been a lot of emphasis on numbers in recent weeks. First in one doctor's office and then another, we pored over statistical data about our newly diagnosed illness.

Among other things, our age is an issue: If we were younger, such and such might have happened; if we were older, just the opposite. At one point we came across charts and graphs showing the possible progression of the disease and our chances for survival. Now all we can think about are odds and probabilities—*How old? How much? How long?*

We certainly want to have general answers to these sorts of questions, and from that standpoint databases and statistics are helpful guidelines. But perhaps now it's time to switch our focus—from *quantity* of life to *quality* of life.

To be sure, it's important to look forward to being around for ten more years, but what about the next ten weeks, ten days, ten hours? How can we best *live* those periods of time? How can we make the most of each day? How can we best thrive rather than merely survive?

THOUGHT FOR TODAY

I will take my mind off the fear of time,
and focus instead on the fullness of time.

July 6

> "In ev'ry storm that either frowns, or falls,
> What an asylum has the soul in prayer!"
>
> EDWARD YOUNG

These days, more than any in the past, we can relate to the axiom "There are no atheists in foxholes." The advent of painful illness and its impact on the family circle has caused us to pray fervently and frequently.

Although we each pray in our own way, according to personal beliefs, the results are similar for all of us. Prayer brings us a sense of stability and also relieves our resentments, obsessions, and fears. By turning to God we are able to renew our hope. We are comforted by the knowledge that God is always at our side and ever-willing to protect and care for us.

Today's difficulties will assuredly be resolved; in God's time, the pain will pass. Peaceful days will return, and the challenges of the present will give way to joy and gratitude.

Will we then remember the rewards of prayer? Will we remember that we can find stability, hope, comfort, strength, guidance, and love not only during times of travail, but at all times?

THOUGHT FOR TODAY

The rewards of prayer are mine
for the asking.

"A man cannot be comfortable
without his own approval."

MARK TWAIN

There was a time when we drew up a daily "to do" list, containing perhaps a dozen or more chores and responsibilities. At day's end we crossed off the ones we had taken care of, and most of the time we felt good about our accomplishments.

The lists have gotten shorter over the last few years. We can't take on as many responsibilities anymore. Even when we complete the few that are on the list, we rarely feel the sense of accomplishment we once did. Sometimes at night we berate ourselves because we "didn't get anything done all day."

Perhaps it's time to stop judging today's accomplishments against yesterday's capabilities. Let's face it—when we are sick and in pain, it can be a formidable undertaking to prepare a meal, vacuum a room, or fold clothes from the dryer.

By the same token, when we are able to handle the relatively small challenges that once didn't warrant a second thought, we ought to give ourselves credit for doing so. By maximizing rather than minimizing our accomplishments in this way, we can enhance our self-worth and begin to feel good about ourselves again.

THOUGHT FOR TODAY

Am I trying to "measure up" against
an outdated yardstick?

July 8

"There is no danger of developing eyestrain from
looking on the bright side of things."
ANONYMOUS

Just about everyone has gone through periods of denial about medical problems, addiction, a deteriorating relationship, or troubling personal problems. We all know about the dangers of denial. When we sidestep, ignore, or otherwise pretend that painful realities don't exist, they usually get worse instead of going away. However, there can be such a thing as "positive denial," especially for people with chronic illness and those who care for them. We've already come to terms with the reality of the illness—its nature and possible course, as well as the toll it is taking—so the issue is no longer acceptance. But acceptance doesn't mean that we have to spend every minute of every day worrying about the illness, dwelling on it, being consumed by it, losing ourselves in it. Positive denial enables us to live a life that goes beyond the realm of pain and illness. It frees us to expand our interests, have a more normal social life, and maintain a self-image unrelated to sickness and caregiving. Positive denial allows us to learn, to laugh, to play, to enjoy friendships and nature—to live.

THOUGHT FOR TODAY

Denial can be positive when it helps
you get on with your life.

"All things are less dreadful
than they seem."
WILLIAM WORDSWORTH

Close friends and family members can sometimes take one look at me and know exactly what kind of a day I'm having, even though I've said nothing at all to them. Chronic pain affects my appearance, there's no question about that. On certain days my drawn face and deep-set eyes clearly indicate the shape I'm in.

Recently, when the dark circles under my eyes were more pronounced than usual, I became quite self-conscious. I even began to wear dark glasses indoors as a disguise of sorts.

That didn't really solve the problem, so I decided to try some makeup. When I nervously described my concern to a cosmetologist in a department store, she began gathering samples of various products. But then she stopped abruptly and said, "I'm going to be really honest with you. There's nothing wrong with your looks. If anything, those shadows give you character. If I were you, I wouldn't do a thing."

I followed her advice, grateful not only for her honesty, but also for the gentle way she helped me realize that my self-perception was awry. What I really needed to work on, I saw, was my self-image, not my appearance.

THOUGHT FOR TODAY

My true reality lies within.

> "Thou tremblest; and the whiteness in thy cheek
> Is apter than thy tongue to tell thy errand."
>
> WILLIAM SHAKESPEARE

We suspected it was cancer and now it's official. The oncologist has reviewed the X-rays and other test results, explaining where the tumor is and how she intends to treat it. She's answered all of our questions, and we have a solid understanding of the situation.

Later, when we are finally alone, panic sets in. A voice within breaks loose and screams, "You have cancer. And you're going to die!" Those despairing words echo for weeks; they rob us of life, exhaust us, and make it almost impossible to pull ourselves together and begin treatment.

Yes, we've all been there. It's one thing to understand a life-threatening illness intellectually, but it's quite another challenge to accept that illness emotionally. Peace of mind comes with total acceptance, which is possible only when the two levels—intellectual and emotional—merge and blend.

It takes time for that to happen—weeks, months, or even longer for some of us. We may have to grieve for the once-healthy bodies we feel we have lost. One way or the other, no matter what we face, we need to talk it out and keep talking it out.

THOUGHT FOR TODAY

Acceptance is far more an emotional and spiritual process than it is an intellectual one.

"If health and a fair day smile upon me,
I am a very good fellow; if a corn trouble my toe,
I am sullen, out of humor, and inaccessible."

MICHEL EYQUEM DE MONTAIGNE

After we had been sick for a while, our relatives gradually opened up about the apprehension they used to feel when they came to visit. "We didn't know who we would spend the afternoon with," they confided, "the nice patient or the evil twin."

Their admissions came as no surprise; by that time we had become quite aware of our emotional ups and downs. More to the point, we could see a direct correlation between our energy swings or pain levels and our disposition.

Now we can pretty much predict our mood and behavior. When we have a lot of energy and are relatively pain-free we laugh easily, smile a lot, and are warm and congenial. On days when we are tired, achy, and feeling sick we tend to be brooding, cranky, and hostile.

We do our best to overcome these illness-generated dark moods; we try hard to be even-tempered and civil with our friends and family members. And since we're not always successful, we're careful not to be hard on ourselves when our disposition gets the best of us and doesn't match our expectations. At such times we give ourselves permission to be alone until the storm has passed.

THOUGHT FOR TODAY

Cut yourself some slack.

"Forsake not God till you
find a better master."
SCOTTISH PROVERB

There was once a catastrophic earthquake in the city where I live. Destruction was widespread and many people were killed, injured, and displaced. Almost immediately, people I know began to wonder, "Is God responsible for this? Is He angry at us?" The city newspaper followed suit and asked local clergy: "Is the earthquake a message from God?"

I used to ask similar questions, and not only in the aftermath of natural disasters or personal calamities; it took very little for me to doubt God's goodness. There came a time, though, when I had to put aside such questions once and for all. The reason, then and now, is that I need God in my life. I need to be able to trust Him completely, no matter what happens to me or around me.

I believe that God is loving, not wrathful. I believe that His power flows in and through our lives as love, continually shaping us and drawing us forward into all that we are capable of being.

I believe that God has a divine plan for each of us, which positively transcends anything we can hope for or even imagine.

THOUGHT FOR TODAY

I choose to believe that God is not punishing and vindictive, but compassionate and loving.

> "At every step the child should be allowed to
> meet the real experiences of life...."
>
> ELLEN KEY

We've all had the experience of being around a loved one who is seriously out of sorts. We sense that something is very wrong, but because the person remains closemouthed and unapproachable, we can't get a handle on it. As a result we feel unsettled, apprehensive, or fearful. We wonder if we've done something wrong. We imagine the worst.

That's exactly how our young children feel when we try to keep our illness a secret, when we pretend that nothing has changed and that everything is all right.

It's natural to want to shield our children from the painful realities of our illness, especially in its prodromal stage—the stage when the forewarning symptoms have produced a diagnosis and we are on an emotional rollercoaster. However, we need to acknowledge the fact that even young children are quite intuitive. They know when the family atmosphere has changed, when something is upsetting their parents. They sense that something is terribly wrong, but they don't actually know what it is.

Because of this, they suffer more from the fear, stress, and even guilt of not knowing than they would if they were told the truth. Clearly, then, the children must be told; we must find a way to be appropriately open and honest about our illness.

THOUGHT FOR TODAY

Truth will brighten the darkness and lessen the fear.

> "Truth is the only safe ground
> to stand upon."
>
> ELIZABETH CADY STANTON

Drastic change is the order of the day around the house, and we can no longer put off telling the children about our illness. But how should we go about it? We want to tell them enough but not too much; we want to answer their questions without raising new ones. We pray that they will be understanding and accepting rather than frightened and insecure.

Before we begin, let's remember that short and simple answers and explanations work best. If a child is given too much information, he or she is likely to feel burdened and helpless.

Timing is critical. Ideally, both parents will participate, and we should pick a time when neither we nor the children are tired or distracted. It's also a good idea to tell all the children at the same time. That way there will be less chance of confusion or misinterpretation. Moreover, if they are together the children will likely reassure each other.

We should try to end the conversation on a note of reassurance and optimism. We might emphasize, for example, that they will always be loved, that their daily needs will be met, and that we are doing everything possible to get well again.

THOUGHT FOR TODAY

Keep it simple, but also keep
it truthful and hopeful.

"How queer everything is to-day! And yesterday things went on just as usual. I wonder if I've been changed in the night? Let me think: was I the same when I got up this morning? I almost think I can remember feeling a little different. But if I'm not the same, the next question is, "Who in the world am I?" Ah, that's the great puzzle."

LEWIS CARROLL

I know a lifeguard who seriously injured his back one summer. The disability kept him off the job for seven months, and he was also unable to participate in the sports—running, swimming, surfing, and karate—that were, in his words, "my whole life."

During the first several weeks off the job my friend was angry, depressed, and practically inconsolable. All he talked about were the things he couldn't do.

When he realized one day that friends and even fellow lifeguards had been giving him a wide berth because of his constant negativity, he became disgusted with his self-pity. "I made up my mind to turn it around, to stop dwelling on what I couldn't do and to begin focusing on what I *could* do," he said.

He gave considerable thought to activities still available to him— not only physical, but also mental and spiritual. He made a list, and worked at it, and soon each day was filled.

My friend's back eventually healed and he was able to resume his demanding lifestyle. However, he told me (and promised himself) he would never forget the simple but profoundly important lesson he had learned while getting well.

THOUGHT FOR TODAY

What will be my focus today—my
incapabilities or my capabilities?

> "We should behave to our friends as we would
> wish our friends to behave to us."
>
> ARISTOTLE

The pain is tolerable today, so you gather your strength for a shopping trip to the mall. Just as you step off the escalator, a former co-worker rushes up and brays, "How *are* you? Oh, you poor thing, we feel so bad for you!" She then takes you by the elbow as if you are a frail ninety-eight-year-old, and nearly trips on your cane as she attempts to guide you to a nearby bench for a chat.

Such encounters can be stressful, uncomfortable, and at times downright humiliating. Fear, discomfort, and similar emotions cause some friends, acquaintances, and even relatives to treat us differently than they did before we became ill. Some are overly solicitous; others talk to us as if we are children; some pretend we are not ill at all, or avoid us.

In many instances we can help the person understand that the illness hasn't changed *who* we are, and that we would appreciate being treated as before. However, when such efforts at communication fail, and we can't bring about understanding or sensitivity, all we can do is work on our own reactions. That's something we can always control.

THOUGHT FOR TODAY

I will take the initiative to
put others at ease.

"The secret of health for both mind and body is
not to mourn for the past, not to worry about the future,
or not to anticipate troubles, but to live in the
present moment wisely and earnestly."

THE BUDDHA

We are learning that there's far more to the healing process than tests, procedures, pills, or any other form of medical treatment. Emotional and spiritual therapies, we believe, are at least equally important. We've already benefited greatly from friendships developed in support groups, from meditation, from activities such as yoga and exercise. How freeing it is when we give ourselves permission to take a healing nap in the middle of the afternoon.

Some of us, however, are not completely comfortable with our new regimen, as beneficial as it is. All too often we feel guilty for spending so much time on ourselves. We wonder if we aren't being self-centered, even narcissistic. Something in our emotional makeup, perhaps arising from childhood admonitions or even adult feelings of unworthiness, restrains us from pursuing the very activities that are essential to our physical, emotional, and spiritual well-being.

But we're fighting such old ideas. We're taking time to uncover, discover, and discard the forces that sometimes turn us into our own worst enemy. After all, our very lives are at stake.

THOUGHT FOR TODAY

I am worthy and fully deserving
of every healing action.

July 18

"Hope, like the short-lived ray that gleams awhile. . .
Cheers e'en the face of misery to a smile."

WILLIAM COWPER

You're back on your feet again, at least for now. You feel well enough, unexpectedly so, to attend your best friend's wedding. One by one or in small groups, the people you know ask how you are doing and how you are feeling.

You tell them the truth, mentioning the chemotherapy, the radiation, and the possibility of another surgery. You let them know how difficult it's been to get through each day. Your friends are sympathetic and try to be upbeat, but you can't help noticing their pained looks, their sadness and disappointment. In addition to the fact that you are uncomfortable with all the attention, you feel terrible for spelling out realities that leave *them* feeling terrible.

Now that it's over you think ahead to the next invitation, the next party. You have two choices. You can avoid such gatherings; on Thanksgiving, Christmas, and New Year's Eve you can shut yourself off from the world and your friends. Or, you can decide well in advance exactly how to respond, what to say, and how to temper the reality of your condition with a high degree of optimism, hopefulness, and faith.

THOUGHT FOR TODAY

Am I sharing my courage as well as my
pain, my faith as well as my fear?

"Most folks are about as happy as they
make up their minds to be."

ABRAHAM LINCOLN

We all know people who have had dramatic personality changes following a catastrophic accident, major surgery, or the onset of serious illness and chronic pain. Some who were once kind, giving, open, and independent are now bitter, abrasive, closed off, and fearful. Then there are those whose attitudes and outlook have been transformed in the opposite way—from recklessness, self-centeredness, and cynicism to stability, humility, and generosity of spirit.

It seems clear, as much from our own experience as the experiences of others, that trauma often positions and primes us for radical change. While we may have very little control over the trauma (the accident, surgery, or illness), we do have a high degree of control, in the form of *choice*, over the ways we change within.

As we move toward healing and wholeness, what choices will we make for ourselves? Will we be judgmental of others, or will we do our utmost to be compassionate? Will we grow stronger and more resilient, or will we see ourselves as frail and vulnerable? Will we be held back by fear or drawn forward by faith?

THOUGHT FOR TODAY

Will my days be shadowed by self-pity
for all that is "bad" or brightened by
gratitude for all that is good?

July 20

"Life is a succession of lessons which
must be lived to be understood."

RALPH WALDO EMERSON

We can read books and attend lectures until our brains are saturated, but neither of these learning methods compares in power and effectiveness to personal experience. This is especially true when the goal is gaining awareness and understanding of our emotional reactions to chronic illness.

Anger and fear are the two emotions that seem to bedevil us most. Periodically (and for many of us, all too regularly) we become angry at the disease, at our bodies for betraying us, and at relapses that follow remissions. We fear that our suffering will worsen, that our doctors don't know what they are doing, and that death lies in wait.

In my own experience with such troubling feelings, I have learned that anger and fear usually arrive hand in hand. Very often I experience and express anger when what I am really feeling is fear.

Perhaps I still believe, as a remnant of childhood, that anger is a more "acceptable" and more "masculine" emotion than fear. It's a problem I need to clarify, because only when I understand my emotional heritage and recognize my feelings for what they truly are, can I confront and work through them.

THOUGHT FOR TODAY

Once I unveil and accept my fears,
they will lose their power to harm me.

"My natural instinct teaches me
(And instinct is important O!)

You're everything you ought to be.
And nothing that you oughtn't O!"

WILLIAM SCHWENK GILBERT

It has been said that there are no boundaries to meditation, and that there are as many ways to meditate as there are people all over the world who do so. Despite this reality, some of us feel self-conscious during meditation. We worry that we are not correctly following the methods recommended in various books or by particular teachers.

The idea that we must closely follow a respected teacher's example (ideally, to the point of exact imitation) is of course contrary to the very spirit of meditation. The primary value of meditation is that it encourages us to be fully ourselves, to gain ever greater awareness and acceptance of who we are.

Teachers and books and tapes can certainly be useful as guidelines, but we are far better off respecting our own inner authority. We are better off trusting our own instincts, wherever they may lead us.

By meditating in our own way rather than someone else's, we gradually gain confidence in ourselves, and learn to heed more readily the urgings of our intuition in *all* areas of life.

THOUGHT FOR TODAY

When it comes to meditation,
my way is the "right" way.

July 22

> "He who lives only to benefit himself confers on
> the world a benefit when he dies."
>
> TERTULLIAN

It would be nice to say that I've finally gotten my willfulness under control, that my feet are firmly planted on the spiritual path, and that I almost always try to seek and do God's will. But unfortunately that's not the case. All too often my various illnesses bring out the worst in me.

At certain times, usually when pain or fever flares, I throw my weight around. The willful child in me wants what he wants when he wants it, and woe betide you if you deny him or stand in his way. Later, when it's clear that things haven't worked out in line with my desires and expectations, I inevitably become disappointed, frustrated, and angry. Also inevitably, my willfulness and self-centeredness activate a host of character defects.

While it's true that my illnesses require me to pay a considerable amount of attention to myself, emotionally as well as physically, that's no excuse to let self-will run riot. Nor is it a license to be manipulative, controlling, or unkind to friends, family, or healthcare professionals. It's certainly not a license to forsake God's will in favor of my own.

THOUGHT FOR TODAY
_____

Self-will is not the solution to my problems
but the cause of them.

"Acceptance of what has happened
is the first step to overcoming the
consequences of any misfortune."

WILLIAM JAMES

Sitting nervously in the doctor's waiting room, your mind wanders back to other waiting rooms, other illnesses, other injuries. When you were twelve you fell off a bike and broke your leg. You were out of action for eight weeks, but luckily the cast came off just in time for summer vacation. Several years later there was that terrible bout of bronchitis, which seemed to drag on forever. Then, when you were thirty, you underwent an emergency appendectomy.

That's the way it used to be. You got sick, then you got well. You injured something and it healed. But this is different. This is a chronic illness, unlike anything you've ever had. There was a beginning, but there's no end in sight. No one has been able to promise that in six weeks, six months, or even six years you will be cured.

Because chronic illness is so different, it requires something entirely different from you. Clearly, patience isn't enough. In order to once again enjoy a rich and rewarding life, you have to now think about changing on the inside—your self-image, your attitudes, your outlook. Now, above all, you have to think about gaining acceptance.

THOUGHT FOR TODAY

Dear God, please help me to
change the things I can.

July 24

> "Circumstances do not make the man,
> they reveal him."
>
> JAMES ALLEN

We may be down, but we're not out. Just because we're sick, that doesn't mean we have to give up a single one of the responsibilities and activities that have always been part of our daily routine. Right?

Many of us feel somehow diminished when illness slows us down. So at first we may try to continue exactly as before, hanging on like a bull rider and praying we don't get hurt when we are thrown.

It's true that much of our self-esteem comes from everyday routines, the things we do for ourselves and others. Yet even though we are ill, we can continue to gain self-esteem in those ways—as long as we go about it differently. We may not be able to do all of the things we used to do, but that doesn't mean we can't be successful in establishing a fulfilling routine.

The key to making a smooth adaptation is planning and strategy. We can learn to work smarter, not harder. We can do some things differently, delegate others, and give up others entirely. We can learn when to spend energy, when to conserve it and, most importantly, how to regain and maintain our independence.

THOUGHT FOR TODAY

Illness does not diminish me
in any way.

"Who knows most, doubts not."
ROBERT BROWNING

Some of us suffer illnesses which are not readily detectable in our outward appearance. Our symptoms fluctuate in severity; we go in and out of remission; even when we are feeling the worst, we sometimes have the rosy-cheeked glow of health. And because we are not obviously impaired, certain people have a hard time believing we are sick.

Some may be so insensitive and bold as to accuse us of "faking it" to avoid responsibility at home or at work. Others may not tell us to our face that they think we are crybabies or hypochondriacs, but they don't have to; their innuendoes speak volumes.

It's hurtful and humiliating to have our honesty questioned in these ways; if we're not prepared, such encounters can be highly stressful. That's why it's important for us to become well-educated about our illnesses. We're then able to knowledgeably and assertively educate friends, co-workers, and relatives who may doubt us.

These days, as the result of our efforts, we rarely have to go on the defensive. The illness itself is challenging enough; we don't have to take on the added burden of proving that we're actually sick.

THOUGHT FOR TODAY

For every person who may doubt my illness, there are dozens who are well informed and supportive.

July 26

> "The mind is free,
> what e'er afflict the man."
>
> MICHAEL DRAYTON

When one of my brothers came to visit, my wife and I decided to prepare a rather elaborate barbecue meal. It's not the sort of thing we do very often, and it turned out to be a lot of fun. Instead of "eating and running" as we frequently do, we lingered at the table.

When we finally did get up and stretch, I realized with surprise that for more than two hours I had been totally unaware of the severe pain that had been plaguing me all that week. Although I didn't know it at the time, I had been experiencing pain relief through distraction.

It may seem all too simple, but the fact is that distraction, by taking our mind off the pain, can indeed provide relief. We can effectively use the distraction technique when we are waiting for pain medication to start working, for example, or by itself to relieve pain when it is relatively mild.

All sorts of activities can be used to distract our attention from pain. In my own case, the diversions that work best include movie- or TV-watching, slow and rhythmic breathing, listening to music through headphones, playing video poker on my computer, or immersing myself in a good book.

THOUGHT FOR TODAY

I will open my mind to new methods of pain relief.

"Every day is an opportunity
to make a new happy ending."
ANONYMOUS

Living in the now is easier said than done, especially when one's life is shadowed by pain and illness. In spite of our determination to appreciate the gift of each new moment, all too often we find ourselves dwelling fearfully in the future or morbidly in the past.

A common problem is that we make advance judgments of what the unfolding moment, or event, or journey, already holds for us. In other words, we allow our ideas, beliefs, and attitudes—the things we think we already "know" about what is going to take place—to distort actuality and keep us from seeing and experiencing things as they really are.

We certainly can't "force" ourselves to live in the now. We can keep in mind, however, that each new moment is unlike any other, containing unique possibilities, challenges, opportunities, and joys.

We can be reminded, moreover, that life is most meaningful when we fully assimilate what is taking place around us. Life is richest when we let our senses guide us; when we feel our feelings and open our minds; when we gain brand-new awarenesses, make new judgments, and enjoy new adventures.

THOUGHT FOR TODAY

I will try to grasp the extraordinariness
of the ordinary.

> "It is not because things are difficult
> that we do not dare, it is because we
> do not dare that things are difficult."
>
> SENECA

If someone asked you to rate the past year on a scale of one to ten, you'd probably give it a two. You've had more sick days then well ones. To make things worse, a whole lot of other things have gone wrong and demanded your attention. You often feel that your illness is quite enough of a burden without any additional difficulties.

Those of us with chronic pain and illness are quite familiar with such feelings. Not surprisingly, therefore, we're sometimes tempted to avoid matters unrelated to our illness. The problem is that when we habitually ignore or try to escape everyday problems and responsibilities, they don't go away. Indeed, they usually multiply and become even more burdensome.

Whether your outside challenges concern finances, legal matters, relationships, or home repairs, you don't have to face them alone. There's bound to be someone in your life who can help. Furthermore, you don't have to resolve all of your problems at the same time, nor do you have to take on an individual problem in its entirety.

THOUGHT FOR TODAY

With a little help, you can accomplish just about anything, a day at a time.

> "'Tis not every question that
> deserves an answer."
>
> THOMAS FULLER

We're embarrassed to say the words aloud, but at times we can't help thinking them: *Why me?* They are discomforting, self-pitying words—in a way, more burdensome than the illness itself.

When we ask the "why me" question, we don't really want an answer. For when the answers do come, from ourselves or others, they are speculative and unsettling: "It was the cigarettes, two packs a day for thirty years." "It was the diet, all that red meat." "It was the perfectionism... the self-loathing... the resentment... the lifestyle..."

For some of us, the answers revolve around different kinds of blame. We blame our parents for damaging our psyches; our doctors for their passivity, self-protectiveness, or ignorance; society for its pollution of the environment. And we may blame God for judging us, punishing us, inflicting the illness upon us.

"Why me?" How tormenting those words can be! As long as we waste our energy searching for nonexistent answers, we hinder our progress toward healing and wholeness. So we must move beyond "why" and focus instead on more relevant questions such as: "What can I learn from this?" "What good can come out of this?" "How can my experience help others?"

I will stop looking for the answer, and perhaps then the question will go away.

July 30

> "A favor well bestowed is almost as great an honor
> to him who confers it as to him who receives it."

RICHARD STEELE

A neighbor and close friend of mine is recovering from a stroke. When I walked by his window one morning, he asked if I could drive him to the bank. I said that I would, and suggested that we also have lunch together.

In the coffee shop, when my friend thanked me for the ride, I told him I was glad he had asked. He smiled, then said, "I'm getting better at that. I finally figured out that people want to help, but they often don't know how. Some of them are probably embarrassed to approach me. So I decided it was up to me to make the first move."

The way he did it, he explained, was to sit down with close friends and relatives and speak freely about his feelings and needs as a recovering stroke patient. "I told them how scared I was right after the stroke. I described the rehab program, especially the speech therapy. And I was able to let them know exactly the kinds of help I need while I'm getting better.

"It was like breaking down a wall," he added. "There's no more embarrassment. It's a lot more comfortable—for everyone."

THOUGHT FOR TODAY
Reaching out sometimes
awaits an invitation.

"Through love, through hope,
and faith's transcendent dower,
We feel that we are greater than we know."
WILLIAM WORDSWORTH

The spirit of healing is abundant in my life. It flourishes within and around me, at this very moment, reflecting God's grace.

I affirm that God's desire for my wellness is unconditional, no less so than His love for me. I need not improve or try to perfect myself in any way to become worthy of wellness. I need not earn healing by changing myself, by finishing that which is unfinished, by coming to terms with past or present difficulties. The stage is already set for healing.

What I can and will do today is develop a vocabulary of healing phrases—*I am energetic and strong; I am blessed; with God, I can.*

I will center my thoughts on wellness and well-being, focusing on faith rather than fear, strength rather than weakness, capability rather than disability. Even though I face health challenges, I will continue to see my body as the true God-given miracle that it is. I will find hope in its exquisite design and function, and its remarkable capabilities for positive change and renewal.

Within me, right now, an amazing synergism is taking place, whereby each muscle, organ, nerve—every single cell—is working harmoniously to heal and restore me.

THOUGHT FOR TODAY

Wellness is my destination;
faith is my vehicle.

August

"It is a strange desire, to seek power, and to lose liberty;
or to seek power over others, and to lose
power over a man's self."

FRANCIS BACON

In our own households as well as in outside circles, some of us were self-appointed managers and controllers. We had specific and usually inflexible ideas of how other people should live their lives, from the foods they ate and cars they drove to how they spent their money and raised their kids. When they didn't go along with our advice and admonitions, we applied pressure.

When we became ill, one of our first concerns was how friends and family members would handle the news. We were more worried about their inability to get along without our "guidance" and involvement than we were about our own diagnosis and prognosis.

Clearly, our priorities were seriously awry, and we soon realized that our need to manage and control others—our codependency—was a serious character flaw requiring immediate attention.

As part of the treatment and recovery process, we came gradually to understand that we could ill-afford to squander precious energy in futile attempts to run other people's lives. In the interest of healing and wholeness, we would have to put ourselves first, in an entirely different way than ever before.

THOUGHT FOR TODAY

Energy spent on unachievable
objectives is energy wasted.

August 2

> "You shall have joy, or you shall have power,
> said God; you shall not have both."
>
> RALPH WALDO EMERSON

When we try to manipulate and control other people we are bound to fail, and to feel often disappointed, frustrated, and angry. It all adds up to a body full of stress, which is the last thing our immune system needs these days. Stress not only compromises our physical health but also exhausts us emotionally.

That's why we are working so hard to accept our powerlessness over others, and to detach ourselves emotionally from them. We know from exasperating experience that we can't "fix" other people, solve their problems, or even make them listen to us.

A major goal today is to give our close friends and family members the opportunity to learn and grow on their own by following their own hearts, making their own decisions, and benefiting from their own mistakes.

This doesn't mean that we've stopped loving our friends and relatives, or that we're no longer attentive and supportive. It simply means that where once we tried to manage the lives of those around us, we've now become willing to step aside and, with love, release them into God's hands.

THOUGHT FOR TODAY

When I release someone with love,
the person I free is myself.

"Trust not to thy feeling, for whatever it be now,
it will quickly be changed into another thing."

THOMAS À KEMPIS

It took me quite a long time to accept each of my illnesses, and longer still to accept all of them together. Several years ago, I finally reached the point where I had truly come to terms with my chronic health problems.

Recently, I realized that my acceptance of the illnesses on a broad scale doesn't necessarily mean that I fully accept the day-to-day ups and downs—the "nitty gritty" of being sick.

If I'm so accepting of my illnesses, I asked myself, why do I get embarrassed when my memory fails? Why do I become angry when I see pain-etched dark circles under my eyes? Why do I still become frustrated and impatient when I lose my breath climbing stairs?

What I'm learning, it seems, is that I get the most benefit from acceptance when I put it into practice each day, in all kinds of situations. In other words, acceptance is not just a principle, but a tool. I can use it to smooth out my ragged emotions when I hate the way I look. And I can use it to restore my perspective when I feel singled out and abandoned.

THOUGHT FOR TODAY

Do I fully accept myself right now,
exactly as I am?

"There is no wealth but life."

JOHN RUSKIN

Because we are so often in pain or preoccupied with other debilitating symptoms, some of us are constantly on the lookout for "windows" in time when we will somehow be pain-free and carefree. We know that when those occasions arrive we will find joy, clarity, and peace. We will take a short vacation from illness and, at least for that interlude, reclaim our lives.

But what about the quality of life in between those windows? Why do we have to reserve joy and serenity only for special times, when everything falls magically into place? Why can't we strive to reclaim our lives on a daily basis?

No matter what our physical condition, there are actions we can take to find joy and peace. Meditation, yoga, and other avenues of self-discovery are always available to us. We can set new goals that relate more to inner healing than to outside pursuits.

To give our lives an ongoing sense of meaning and purpose, we can remain committed to spiritual growth. We can try to live by spiritual principles, and to strengthen our relationship with God. And just as His presence makes a difference in our life, we can try each day to make a difference in the lives of others.

THOUGHT FOR TODAY

I can begin to reclaim my life right now.

"Sweet is pleasure after pain."

JOHN DRYDEN

We often talk about pain in my cancer-survivors support group. Several months ago a member expressed concern that her cancer would recur, then admitted how frightened she was of the devastating and uncontrollable pain that might accompany it.

Everyone in the room related to those fears. Soon, several of us pointed out that the cancer had not recurred and probably never would; that the pain had not yet arrived and probably never would; but that the fear was already eating her up and causing pain of another kind.

The discussion that night was quite hopeful and encouraging. There were ten of us, as I recall, and we each described from personal knowledge or experience a variety of advances in pain management. We talked about all sorts of effective new techniques, from implantable morphine pumps and nerve-deadening injections to patches that slowly release pain-killing drugs through the skin, as well as numerous nontraditional medicines and approaches.

We also took comfort from our awareness that the medical profession is paying a lot more attention to the pain of patients these days. Doctors have begun to fully understand, more promptly and pragmatically, that pain *needs* to be controlled and *can* be controlled.

THOUGHT FOR TODAY

Fear of pain can be more
agonizing than actual pain.

"There never was night that had no morn."

DINAH MULOCK CRAIK

Who would have thought that seriously ill people could one day be given new life through heart, liver, lung, or kidney transplants?

Who would have thought that a new medical science, psychoneuroimmunology, would rapidly expand the frontiers of mind-body healing, teaching us how to influence our immune systems positively?

Who would have thought that the power of lasers could be refined to perform delicate eye surgery, or to vaporize life-threatening arterial blockages?

Who could have imagined that computer-designed, electronically driven prostheses would dramatically improve the capabilities of people who are severely challenged by injury or disease?

Who would have thought that certain forms of cancer, once deemed incurable, could be successfully treated with massive doses of radiation, or chemotherapy?

Who could have imagined tools and technologies—such as magnetic resonance imaging, or computerized tomography—that would allow physicians to locate and diagnose illness or injury without performing invasive surgery?

Who would have thought that Human Genome Project scientists would be so far along in mapping DNA, pinpointing the location of genes that can predispose people to serious disease?

THOUGHT FOR TODAY

Where there is life there is hope.
Where there is hope there is life.

"What soon grows old?
Gratitude."
ARISTOTLE

Those of us who had been gravely ill and then came back, so to speak, were afterward infused with a profound sense of gratitude. We had been forced to face the actual possibility of our own death, and that caused us to look at our lives in an entirely new way. Then and there we became sharply aware of what *really mattered*. As survivors we saw each new day of life as a precious gift.

Initially, that extraordinary experience strengthened our spiritual core and reshaped our perspective. But the passage of time and the exigencies of daily living now presents us with continuing choices. We can allow gratitude to fade from the forefront of our consciousness. By making that choice, we again take life for granted, and slip into self-pity at the first hint of adversity.

The other choice, of course, is to use the near-death experience as a catalyst for ongoing positive change. When we begin to feel sorry for ourselves, when minor inconveniences begin to seem catastrophic, we revisit and renew the gratitude we have gained as survivors. We revere this life, this day, this moment.

THOUGHT FOR TODAY

Thank God for this precious day.

August 8

> "The heart benevolent and kind
> The most resembles God."
>
> ROBERT BURNS

It's only 2:00 p.m. but it feels like midnight. The X-rays were taken at the east end of town, the blood tests at the west end, and the doctor's appointment was way out in the suburbs. You are frazzled and exhausted, but at least you're finally home.

So what are you going to do for the rest of the day? Are you going to rerun the morning's events and relive the stress? Are you going to call up your best friend and complain? Are you going to dwell sorrowfully on the dark shadows under your eyes, and chastise yourself for getting sick in the first place?

How about being kind to yourself? Instead of frowning into the mirror and telling yourself you look horrible, why not do some nice things for your body and spirit? Take a warm bath, schedule a hair appointment or a color consultation.

Instead of trying to wind down by overeating or drinking, choose positive ways to release tension. Enjoy a delicious, nutritious meal. Get some exercise if you are able, or take a nice long nap.

Why not reflect on all the progress you've made, not only physically but emotionally and spiritually? Why not give yourself the credit you deserve?

THOUGHT FOR TODAY

Not just on this difficult day, but every day
I will try to be kind to myself.

August 9

> "Time discovers truth."
>
> SENECA

A few summers ago, while traveling through the Yucatan Peninsula in Mexico, I missed a bus and had to wait three hours for the next one. I claimed one of the few remaining seats in the crowded, noisy waiting room and began to stare at the wall clock directly in front of me.

The crowd grew, the temperature rose, the odors intensified, and my discomfort escalated. The one thing that didn't advance was time itself; the hands of the clock seemed frozen in place.

Nothing slows a clock like discomfort, and nothing stops time altogether like pain. Thankfully, however, there is a corollary: *Nothing speeds up time like keeping busy.*

I could have done many things to ease my discomfort and help the time pass that hot afternoon in the Yucatan. I could have read, worked a crossword puzzle, written postcards, or struck up a conversation and practiced my Spanish.

The same choice is available to me these days when I am in pain. I can focus on the nature and intensity of that pain, along with the grindingly slow passage of time. Or I can occupy myself with various alternatives, from creative pursuits to spiritual ones.

THOUGHT FOR TODAY

Will it be time endured or time spent?

"My hopes are not always realized,
but I always hope."

OVID

When doctors decided on an intensive course of chemotherapy for a friend of mine with cancer, she considered the expected side effects a small price to pay for the prospect of getting well again. As it turned out, the treatment was ineffective, and the side effects were far worse than anyone had anticipated. My friend was not only frustrated and disillusioned, but furious. She felt that her doctors, the hospital and, indeed, medicine as a whole had failed her.

Many of us have had similar experiences. Because of well-publicized successes in pharmacology and medicine, and because we so desperately want (and need) new drugs and treatments to work in our lives, we tend to exaggerate their potential capabilities. When they don't work as well as we had hoped—or if they don't work at all—the gap between our expectations and reality causes us to lose faith and become cynical and angry.

Unfortunately, medicine is not always an exact science. For all the spectacular successes, there are few cures for the illnesses that claim the most lives. That's why all of us—patients and caregivers alike—must try to temper our hopeful expectations with objectivity and realism.

THOUGHT FOR TODAY

I will ground my faith and hope
on the bedrock of reality.

"No passion so effectually robs the mind of all its powers of acting and reasoning as fear."

EDMUND BURKE

When my wife found me sitting cross-legged on the couch, she knew immediately that something was wrong. My skin was ashen and damp, and I looked fearful and confused.

She questioned me, in a gentle and roundabout sort of way, trying to determine whether my condition warranted a trip to the emergency room or simply a calming heart-to-heart talk. She knows from experience that strange or painful new symptoms sometimes cause me to panic.

This was one of those times. I had awakened with unusual muscular spasms in my chest. My mind immediately exaggerated the symptom's severity and convinced me that I was on the verge of cardiac arrest. When my wife realized that my fear had taken me captive, she was able to "talk me down."

Of course, we can't always count on a spouse, partner, or caregiver being around when panic strikes. We have to learn how to deal with these episodes of irrationality in other ways. We can call the doctor, just to be on the safe side. We can make an effort to treat the symptom or lessen the pain. And we can become involved in an activity, so as to divert our mind and free ourselves from its clutches.

THOUGHT FOR TODAY

Panic rarely reflects reality.

August 12

"A healthy mind has an easy breath."
ANONYMOUS

We've done it thousands upon thousands of times a day, every day, from the very moment of birth. We've done it involuntarily, usually without thought or even awareness, and it has kept us alive. *Breathing*.

Because we take breathing for granted, we tend to overlook its value as a multipurpose tool in our pursuit of wellness. To begin with, we can use our breathing power to counteract some of the debilitating effects of illness. When fatigue or muscle soreness turns even the simplest chore into a major challenge, deep and rhythmic breathing oxygenates the blood, revitalizes the muscles, and provides a burst of new energy.

Deep, steady breathing can also be an effective stress reducer. By consciously focusing on our breathing, we can divert our mind from flights of fury and similar self-destructive journeys.

When we find ourselves fearfully projecting backward or forward in time—when we're angry, resentful, anxious, or impatient—we can return to the here and now and regain a measure of serenity by tuning in once again to our breathing.

THOUGHT FOR TODAY

Breathing makes it possible for us to live, but it also helps us to achieve poise, patience, and tranquility.

> "Our life is what our
> thoughts make it."
>
> MARCUS AURELIUS

Most of my friends know that I suffer from an illness that fluctuates in severity. Consequently, hardly a day goes by when someone doesn't ask me, "How do you feel?" I'm grateful for their concern, of course, but it recently occurred to me that a more appropriate question might be, "How do you *think?*" I say this because the way I think profoundly influences the way I feel.

Let's say, for example, that I awaken to the unmistakable sound of Santa Ana winds gusting to forty miles per hour. If I focus obsessively on how the low humidity and swirling dust will dry my skin and wreck my sinuses, I guarantee myself a highly stressful day, during which every ache and pain will be larger than life. If, on the other hand, I make up my mind this time to ignore the seasonal weather phenomenon and keep busy indoors, I'm likely to have a decent day.

It's easy to forget that the way I think pretty much determines how I feel. Yet each and every day I face dozens of situations inviting attitudinal choices. If I choose to think about an event or circumstance in a positive rather than a negative way, it is likely that I will have a satisfying and even pleasurable experience.

THOUGHT FOR TODAY

I choose to be optimistic,
hopeful, and grateful.

August 14

> "When our perils are past, shall our gratitude sleep?
> No,—here's to the pilot that weathered the storm!"
>
> GEORGE CANNING

Visiting hours are over, but one woman remains at her husband's bedside in the ward. We can't make out what she is saying, but we can hear the soothing tone of her voice and we can almost feel the reassuring touch of her hand. At that moment we begin thinking about all the people in our lives, over the years and to this day, who have been comforting, encouraging, loving, and selfless.

A wave of gratitude sweeps through us as we remember these special people. There were those who refused to give up on us when, as young adults, we got into serious trouble. There was the mother, the father, the sister, the dear friend who helped us regain a sense of self-worth. And there are the treasured friends and relatives who, last week, yesterday, and just several hours ago smoothed the bed sheets, brushed our hair, and assuaged our fears.

As night falls we thank God for these special people. In our prayers we let Him know that we deeply appreciate who they are and how they have come to us, and especially the fact that each bears witness of His abiding love for every one of His children.

THOUGHT FOR TODAY

In my life, God works through people.

"The pain of the mind is worse than
the pain of the body."

PUBLILIUS SYRUS

Pain is such a private thing, so intensely personal and difficult to put into words. When it strikes or flares anew, we are hard-pressed to pinpoint its location or articulate its intensity.

But the doctor needs to know and we do our best. "Does it hurt here?" he asks, prodding gingerly. "That's probably it," we reply, embarrassed at our waffling. "What does it feel like?" he asks. And though it hurts like the devil at that very moment, we are completely tongue-tied.

Later, on the way to the pharmacy, we are frustrated at our inability to make clear to someone else what remains agonizingly clear to ourselves. We are annoyed at our failure to come even close to describing the where, when, and how of our pain. And that's really the thing about pain; it frequently defies description entirely.

Yet we do have our moments. Among the more joyous human connections are those that take place when two or more people share the same illness and the same kind of pain, and are able to communicate without the burden of description or simply by uttering the words, "Oh, yes, I know!"

THOUGHT FOR TODAY

Don't compound the pain by focusing
on your inability to describe it.

August 16

"What you think of yourself is much more important
than what others think of you."

SENECA

It's time to tell a few close friends about the illness, but we're
reluctant to do so. We feel awkward and anxious, as if we've done
something wrong. We have the disturbing sense that we're no longer
equal to others, but instead somehow "less than." We feel broken and
alienated. For a brief moment, we wonder guiltily if we've brought
this whole thing on ourselves and somehow deserve it.

Such dangerous and destructive feelings rob us not only of physical
and emotional health, but also of any sense of well-being we may have
developed over the years. That's why it's so important to confront
these feelings as soon as they arise.

We can remind ourselves that self-doubt of this sort is frequently
triggered by old ideas which have nothing to do with today's realities.

We can remind ourselves that illness truly is a natural part of life,
contrary to societal pressures that would have us believe otherwise.

Finally, we can remind ourselves that in essence we are the same as we
ever were, except for one thing: Because we are learning to transcend
illness, we are becoming stronger and ever more courageous.

THOUGHT FOR TODAY

When negative feelings about myself surface,
I will not take them to heart.

> "Memory, of all the powers of the mind,
> is the most delicate and frail."
>
> BEN JONSON

A year or so ago I started becoming uncharacteristically forgetful. I wouldn't remember the plot of a movie I'd seen the week before. I would go marketing and forget the most important item. I'd miss a bill payment deadline. I became most upset, and even alarmed, when I occasionally forgot conversations I'd had with my wife.

My first reaction was to be harshly self-critical; I'd shake my head and silently curse myself for being stupid. As one can imagine, this approach did little to improve my memory but quite a lot to erode my self-esteem.

I've gradually come to understand that chronic illness, and especially its accompanying pain, can be extremely distracting. The physical and emotional tensions brought on by illness have distinctly negative effects on our thought and memory processes. Memory also suffers when we are fatigued, fearful, or preoccupied with ourselves.

What I've learned to do on the "bad days" is lighten up and not expect so much from my memory. List-making is of course essential. And, to enhance my self-esteem, I try to give myself credit for all the things I remember, instead of deprecating myself for the things I sometimes forget.

THOUGHT FOR TODAY

Not just on the good days, but every day, I will respect myself.

August 18

"Much unhappiness has come into the world because of bewilderment and things left unsaid."

FYODOR MIKHAYLOVICH DOSTOYEVSKY

You've been housebound and alone for two days now. Your husband is involved in a tennis tournament, and his friends have called repeatedly for information about the event. You have been less than friendly, if truth be told.

Because your illness prevents you from participating in certain activities that were once a big part of your life together, you sometimes feel sorry for yourself. You used to play tennis too, and now you feel left out, not to mention resentful and jealous.

It's normal for chronically ill people to have such feelings. If given free rein, however, strong negative emotions such as self-pity, resentment, and jealousy can cause physical harm, and also severely strain intimate relationships.

The starting point for resolution is open and honest communication. It may be necessary for you to clarify your needs, and for your partner or spouse to do the same. By putting pride aside and telling each other with sensitivity exactly how you each feel, you will be able to achieve better understanding, mutual accommodation, and renewed closeness.

THOUGHT FOR TODAY

Have I let it be known *why* I'm out of sorts?

"Bad habits are like a comfortable bed,
easy to get into, but hard to get out of."
PROVERB

As we know full well, the advent of illness brings countless changes to our lives. At times it seems that everything familiar has been turned inside out and upside down, from how we eat, sleep, and get around to the way we interact with others.

As weeks and then months go by, some of these changes bring about new patterns of living. We can learn a lot from such patterns, so it can be extremely useful to identify and understand our new ways of thinking, feeling, and acting.

Some patterns work to our advantage; they lead to heightened self-acceptance and self-esteem, and feelings of well-being. Those are the patterns we want to keep. Other patterns are harmful; they cause stress, self-deprecation, tension in relationships, and also threaten our physical health. Those are the patterns we want to modify or eliminate.

Very often, patterns develop without our knowledge. However, once we become aware of their existence, and take the time to evaluate the effects they are having on our physical and emotional health—we can gain control and exercise our power of choice.

THOUGHT FOR TODAY

Patterns can be teachers.

August 20

"If I were to begin life again, I should want it as it was.
I would only open my eyes a little more."

JULES RENARD

I recently became aware of a seemingly harmless behavioral pattern, which actually had been causing me to feel worse than usual. I had gotten into the habit of eating very little for breakfast. As a result, by midmorning I would become shaky and have difficulty concentrating. The solution was simple and obvious: Go back to preparing a nutritious breakfast or have a snack before lunch.

Such discoveries may not seem like much to those who enjoy good health, but they can make quite a difference to people like myself who are challenged by chronic illness. By becoming aware of health-related living patterns, I can avoid costly detours on my journey toward healing and wellness. For example, when I fall into a pattern of dependency on others to do things for me that are actually within my capability, I invariably feel "less than" and guilty.

At the positive end of the scale, a pattern of early morning exercise or meditation almost always brings on a sense of accomplishment and well-being that stays with me throughout the day. Similarly, my pattern of support-network involvement helps me turn feelings of alienation and self-pity into ones of connectedness and hopefulness.

THOUGHT FOR TODAY

What can I do to preempt the harmful patterns,
and preserve the helpful ones?

"The comforter's head never aches."

ITALIAN PROVERB

We don't like to use the word, or even to acknowledge the emotion, but many of us with chronic illness can be quite needy at times. We need to vent our frustrations and fears. We need to be understood, to be comforted. We need advice and reassurance.

For the most part our families are there for us. They do their very best to meet our needs even when they are fearful and exhausted themselves.

What a relief it is—for everyone involved—when we join a support group. Our family members no longer have to be on emotional call every minute of the day. We can tell, just by the expressions on their faces that the pressure is off. As for ourselves, we've found a way to meet the emotional demands of our illness without feeling guilty about it.

What a Godsend it is to be involved with others who share the same illness and therefore understand exactly what we go through. There's a powerful new healing force in our lives: Support groups provide not only fellowship and the deepest possible understanding, but also real solutions to real needs.

THOUGHT FOR TODAY

Let us grow, let us heal—together.

August 22

> "In ourselves, In our own honest hearts and
> chainless hands, Will be our safeguard."
>
> THOMAS NOON TALFOURD

As we saw it, one of the hallmarks of maturity was the fact that we were "okay" with ourselves. That is to say, we had a high degree of self-acceptance; we were comfortable with who we were, what we had achieved, how far we had come, and where we were headed.

Illness has caused us to look at self-acceptance in an entirely new way. Where once being "okay with ourselves" flowed mainly from our accomplishments—as skilled athletes, good parents, successful entrepreneurs, or talented creators—it now flows primarily from our inner selves.

Today self-acceptance means honoring and valuing ourselves exactly as we are right now. It is in no sense a concession that we'll never be able to return to our old life, or become what we once hoped to be.

Self-acceptance means acknowledging and accepting every bit of ourselves. It includes not only the physical changes that have taken place for better or worse, but also the very special and enduring qualities—such as our capacity for understanding, empathy, and love—that reflect our true essence.

THOUGHT FOR TODAY

Do I accept only the seemingly "good things" about myself?

"God heals and the
doctor takes the fee."

BENJAMIN FRANKLIN

We all know how frustrating, discouraging, and, yes, *infuriating* it is to buck the bureaucracy; to search out lost records and misplaced lab results; to weigh contradictory advice; to be confronted by discourteous doctors and nurses; and to be subjected, sometimes unnecessarily, to batteries of painful and expensive tests. The medical system—what a nightmare it can be!

But we are finding pathways through the maze; we're making the system work for us. Primarily, we're becoming educated about our illnesses so that we can assertively ask knowledgeable questions and insist on understandable answers. We're also trying to be more appreciative of overworked and dedicated healthcare professionals who are trapped in their own parts of the system.

Yet even with the progress we're making, we still can be swept along by other patients' negative attitudes. It's sometimes all too tempting to assume a "victim" mentality, to condemn everything and everyone in the medical system, to become bitter and resentful.

But we are working on that, too. We know full well that such a frame of mind hurts no one but ourselves.

THOUGHT FOR TODAY

How can I help them to help me?

August 24

> "You will soon break the bow if
> you keep it always stretched."
>
> PHAEDRUS

Relax. It's a good word, a healing action, a comforting feeling. When I relax I not only help myself but also those around me. Everyone benefits—family, friends, doctors, nurses. Frowns turn to smiles, laughter comes easily; we're back on the same wavelength.

I used to think that one could relax only by doing nothing, by being completely inactive. I've since come to realize that I can relax even when I'm deeply involved in an activity. That's because relaxation is as much a state of mind as it is a physical release of stress and tension.

There are, of course, many avenues to relaxation and each of us has familiar and favorite ones, from music and artwork to exercise and meditation. Personally, I have found that one of the most effective ways to relax is through prayer. Some days I set aside time to "talk" with God, and afterwards I almost always feel centered and peaceful again.

Prayer can be especially comforting when I face tumultuous or challenging situations. In order to free and relax myself at such times, I focus my thoughts on God's presence and power within and around me. It works, it truly does.

THOUGHT FOR TODAY

Relaxation begins in my mind.

> "It is easy when we are in prosperity to
> give advice to the afflicted."
>
> AESCHYLUS

First you received flowers. Then you received get well cards, dozens of them. Now that you're home from the hospital you have begun to receive something far more difficult to accept. Relatives, friends, and even acquaintances are bombarding you with unsolicited advice.

You ought to try acupuncture. My uncle has this fabulous orthopedist. Keep your leg elevated. You shouldn't be taking that kind of medication. You should definitely see a specialist.

It's hard to be angry with them because you know they mean well, even though they sometimes become annoyed when you don't take their suggestions. The fact remains, however, that dealing with unsolicited advice is often frustrating, stressful, and confusing.

The thing is, you went to great lengths to find the right healthcare team, and you're committed to their recommendations. The last thing you need is to have your confidence undermined; it's vital for you to approach the treatment plan with assurance, faith, and positive expectations.

When unsolicited advice comes your way, what you can do is listen patiently and open-mindedly. What you can't do—what you should not do—is feel guilty when you choose not to follow the advice.

THOUGHT FOR TODAY

Thanks for your concern, but
I'm already in good hands.

> "The soul is kissed by God
> in its innermost regions."
>
> HILDEGARDE OF BINGEN

For a good part of our lives, many of us have sought fulfillment through our relationships with people, places, and things. We feel fulfilled when we find a new friend or develop a close partnership with someone special. We find fulfillment in certain activities— preparing and savoring an excellent meal, winning a game, displaying our talents and proving our capabilities.

Although such involvements and pursuits enrich our lives, the sense of fulfillment we gain from them frequently does not last. In time, usually a relatively short time, we realize that something important is still lacking.

We have discovered that the truest, deepest, and most lasting sense of fulfillment comes from within ourselves. It flows from our spiritual nature, and the practice of such principles as kindness, tolerance, gratitude, service, and love.

That being the case, fulfillment is always within reach. It matters not whether we are wealthy or destitute, surrounded by others or alone, sick or well. By nurturing and expressing our spiritual selves through thoughts, actions, and conscious contact with God, we can always find true satisfaction and enduring fulfillment.

THOUGHT FOR TODAY

I can find what I need by turning
inward rather than outward.

"I know myself better
than any doctor can."

OVID

There's no question that our attitudes and reactions have profound effects on the healing process. It's become quite clear that negative emotions such as guilt or anger are self-destructive, while positive attitudes and behavior are life-enhancing.

How can we best apply this principle to daily life? How can we observe and possibly influence the way our emotions actually affect our physical selves? The key is vigilant self-awareness, through which we can become increasingly conscious of our thoughts and feelings, and their real-time impact on our bodies.

The next time fear takes over, for example, try to pay close attention to your physical reactions. You'll probably find that a wide spectrum of changes takes place all at once. Adrenaline surges, your heart races, muscles tighten; blood vessels dilate, perspiration flows, your breathing becomes rapid and shallow.

In the same way, carefully observe how your body responds when you cultivate positive thoughts and emotions such as optimism, gratitude, joy, and enthusiasm. It's more than likely that you will be physically limber and relaxed; that tension and pain will diminish; and that you will be enriched with a deep sense of serenity and wellbeing.

THOUGHT FOR TODAY

Keen self-awareness can open the
door to healing changes.

> "The drowning man is
> not troubled by rain."
>
> PROVERB

When someone says they are burned-out, we know exactly what they mean. We've been there ourselves many times, and perhaps feel that way right now. *Burned out, frazzled, fried*—whatever the term we use, it comes down to the same thing.

These phrases are descriptive, to be sure, but they don't really get to the heart of the matter. Expressing ourselves in such a way, without going further, may prevent us from realizing that we're actually experiencing a combination of feelings. And those feelings can be dealt with only if we identify and try to understand them one by one.

When we say we are burned-out, we may really be saying that we're tired, out of shape, and out of energy—and need to get more sleep, more exercise, more nourishment. We may really be saying that we're feeling alienated and disconnected, fearful about the future, and out of control—and need to regain perspective by confiding in a close friend.

When we use terms like burnout, we may really be saying that we've lost all of our patience and much of our hope, and that it's time to turn again to God for the courage to go on.

THOUGHT FOR TODAY
_____

What am I really feeling?

"Two things control men's nature,
instinct and experience."

PASCAL

For several weeks in a row a young woman in my lupus support group complained bitterly about the way her rheumatologist had been treating her. The woman—we'll call her Jan—detailed a litany of rude and inconsiderate behavior ranging from two-hour-long appointment delays to verbal abuse about her weight.

Every one of us felt that Jan should look for a different doctor, one who would be not only knowledgeable but also understanding and caring. No one deserved to be treated as she had been treated; that was a given. An equally important consideration, we all agreed, was the matter of *control*. Chronic illness wrests control from us in so many areas that it's essential to hang on to it or do what's necessary to regain it whenever that becomes possible.

A month passed before Jan was able to find a new doctor, and to work up the courage to tell her abusive rheumatologist why she was firing him. When she announced her accomplishment to the group, she was elated, and we congratulated her. She affirmed, for each of us, that no matter how sick we are, we can assert ourselves to do what's best for our physical, mental, and emotional health.

THOUGHT FOR TODAY

There are always choices and decisions I can make, and actions I can take, to help myself.

"In nature there's no blemish but the mind;
None can be called deformed but the unkind."
WILLIAM SHAKESPEARE

No matter how knowledgeable and sophisticated we are about our medical conditions, there are times when embarrassment about certain symptoms causes us to feel and act like adolescents. It's hard not to be self-conscious when it becomes necessary to reveal and discuss problems which we consider to be private and highly personal.

When such embarrassment causes us to ignore or even deny certain symptoms, we put ourselves at risk in several ways. For one thing, embarrassment and worry are high-stress emotions, and as we well know, even relatively low levels of stress can adversely affect our health. Perhaps more important, we may be covering up and neglecting a symptom that is more serious than we realize.

One way to loosen the grip of self-consciousness is to think about and even visualize the literally hundreds of patients our doctor deals with day in and day out. There is nothing our doctor hasn't seen or heard; he or she understands and respects the human body in every aspect and is certainly not going to judge us because we are having a "personal" problem. Another way to become less self-conscious is to remember that it's not what our body looks like that makes us ugly or beautiful, it's what we do and how we treat others that makes us beautiful or ugly.

THOUGHT FOR TODAY

Admitting my feelings of embarrassment to the doctor will smooth the way for both of us.

"It is not death or hardship that is a fearful thing,
but the fear of hardship and death."

EPICTETUS

The specter of financial insecurity is familiar to anyone who is seriously ill. For example, those of us without medical insurance face a steady depletion of whatever financial resources we may have. Those of us fortunate enough to have insurance must deal with increased premiums, deductibles and co-payments, lower annual limits, and the prospect of cancellation.

Then, too, illness can bring about short work weeks or an inability to work at all, and subsequent loss of income in the face of extraordinary new expenses. The burdens can be overwhelming.

On top of all those heart-wrenching realities—the swift outflow of dollars, the clamor of creditors, the need to declare bankruptcy— there is another problem that brings with it sleepless nights and its very own knot in the gut: the *fear* of financial insecurity.

What do we actually fear? We fear losing something or everything we have. We fear not getting the one thing or all the things we want.

Most of the time, we're limited in what we can do about the money part. But there's certainly a great deal we can do about the fear.

THOUGHT FOR TODAY

My real security can be found in faith.

September

September 1

> "How strong an influence
> works in well-placed words."
> GEORGE CHAPMAN

Illness often breeds sensitivity. In my own case, when I'm in the midst of a flare-up, I tend to take things the wrong way. Recently, for example, when my wife joked that I was "out to lunch," I became angry and sulked for hours.

We relearned an important lesson that day: Each of us must take responsibility for the quality of our own emotional life, regardless of the ups and downs of illness. This responsibility, or the lack of it, is reflected in the way we talk to each other, and especially in the language we use.

One good way to refine communication skills along these lines is to consciously turn "you" statements into "I" statements. That way we're able to express our feelings more considerately and also take personal responsibility for them. To someone who is fragile or defensive because he is ill, for example, there is a huge difference between being told "You're out to lunch" and *I get the feeling that it's hard for you to concentrate today."*

As another example, feelings are far less likely to be hurt when the statement "You make me feel so helpless when you're in pain" is rephrased as *"I wish I could do more to help you feel better."*

THOUGHT FOR TODAY

Am I blaming my feelings
on someone else?

September 2

"Knowing is not enough; we must apply.
Willing is not enough; we must do."

JOHANN WOLFGANG VON GOETHE

Many of the perplexing pressures in our lives these days are beyond our control. Much of what is occurring—from fevers that flare and cells that overrun their boundaries, to joints that stiffen and pain that enslaves—is truly unavoidable.

But what about the pressures we create ourselves? Perhaps we are stubbornly refusing to let go of a relationship that is destructive to all concerned. If so, there is no better time than now to step back for a truly objective view and then take action to set ourselves free.

Perhaps, too, we are attempting to accomplish something that is not within our present capability; or perhaps we have taken on responsibilities that were never meant for us. If so, let's release ourselves from the need to be successful in these undertakings.

We may be trying to overcome personal difficulties through sheer force of will, and as a result those difficulties have been mounting rather than subsiding. If so, today is an ideal day to seek God's guidance and allow ourselves to be led in a different direction.

THOUGHT FOR TODAY

I will try to accept the things I cannot change,
and to change the things I can.

> "Be vigilant, guard your mind
> against negative thoughts."
>
> THE BUDDHA

You don't really know who they are, what they do, where they came from, or how they got so smart. What you do know is that *they* always have had a major impact on your life. These days, more than ever, the invisible *they* are capable of influencing many of your thoughts, decisions, and actions.

Your doctor has given you reason to be optimistic, but *they* say that few people recover from this form of cancer.

The chemotherapy technician thinks there won't be any hair loss with the new combination of drugs, but *they* say you should start shopping for wigs now.

The social services people have encouraged you to continue working as long as you feel up to it, but *they* say it's better to quit your job now before it gets too stressful or embarrassing.

You've been feeling much better and you sense that you are winning the battle, but *they* say you shouldn't get your hopes up.

Who *are* these people? Why are you listening to them and taking their admonitions as gospel? Is it because they are so loud and insistent? Well, that's hardly surprising, since *they* are the voices of fear, discouragement, despair, and defeat.

THOUGHT FOR TODAY

Listen only to the voices of love,
hope, and faith.

September 4

"Each day the world is born anew
For him who takes it rightly."

JAMES RUSSELL LOWELL

When I'm with a gathering of friends and several of them ask me how I've been feeling, I usually answer, simply, "I have good days and not-so good days. Right now I'm doing fine."

I choose that response not only to reduce the pressure on myself (and my friends), but also because it reflects one of the most significant realities of my various illnesses and of lupus in particular.

Since it's difficult to predict which days will be the "good ones," I've committed myself to making the most of them when they come along. When I wake up pain-free and full of energy, I take advantage of the opportunity by riding my bike, going on a short hike and picnic, gardening, going fishing, or cruising a mall with dinner and a movie afterward.

It's a lot harder to feel sorry for myself when I've been able to enjoy life in so many ways on those special days. Also, when a "not-so-good" day comes along and perhaps I have to stay in bed, it doesn't seem quite so bad.

THOUGHT FOR TODAY

Seize the day.

"Harmony makes small things grow;
lack of it makes great things decay."

SALLUST

Shaky relationships can be destroyed by chronic illness, and even idyllic ones can be jeopardized. The stresses of pain and illness often cause simmering conflicts to erupt, and can easily bring about new tensions. We find ourselves dealing with intense and sometimes unfamiliar emotions—rage, dread, alienation. We are forced to cope with uncertainty and exhaustion, not to mention stressful changes in roles and routines.

Under such circumstances, it's necessary for both partners to do everything possible to reduce friction and preserve the peace. One of the best ways to accomplish this is by carefully "choosing battles." For example, the caregiver may at times choose to withhold criticism of the sick person, or to overlook his or her irritating behavior.

Similarly, the one who is ill may decide that past conflicts are no longer worth the struggle, and that even certain long-held "principles," simply aren't important enough to argue about.

Choosing battles should not be thought of as "giving in" or "giving up." Rather, the practice offers a positive way to reestablish teamwork, harmony, and love.

THOUGHT FOR TODAY

How can I minimize conflict? Flexibility, tolerance, and forgiveness are good starting points.

September 6

"It may seem a strange principle to enunciate
as the very first requirement in a Hospital that
it should do the sick no harm."

FLORENCE NIGHTINGALE

You are going back into the hospital for more treatment, and you're dreading it. Your last hospital experience was a nightmare. Besides the usual problems of noise, confusion, and long waits, some nurses didn't seem to understand how much pain you were having, and that it's possible to look fairly normal on the outside and still be in agony.

There are steps you can take to make this stay a better one. First, discuss your pain in advance. Describe to your nurses what the pain is like, its causes, and the control techniques that have worked to relieve it.

Next, do your best to be reasonable and patient. Doctors, nurses, and other members of your team are as human as you are, so try to make allowances for occasional insensitivity or forgetfulness. However, if unsatisfactory performance threatens your well-being, speak up—calmly but assertively. Straightforward communications are far more effective than angry demands or temper tantrums.

Finally, don't spare the compliments for a job well done. Let nurses and other staffers know how much you appreciate their efforts to keep you comfortable and help you get well.

THOUGHT FOR TODAY

Hospitals aren't hotels, but there are things I can say and do to make my stay more comfortable.

"I have not appreciated what You have done for me,
Lord; I take from others and exploit them.
What face shall I show You, Lord?"

GRANTH SAHIB

There have been times in the past when I "exploited" one or another of my illnesses. I usually did so to get my way, to avoid doing something unpleasant but necessary, or to excuse my own unkind behavior.

Looking back, I recall always feeling guilty and uncomfortable following such episodes, as if I had stolen something from someone without their knowledge. Of course, I was the real victim.

Each time I pleaded "exhaustion" to get out of a social obligation or to extend a deadline, I eroded my self-esteem. Each time I exaggerated my pain to manipulate somebody into doing something I could have done for myself, I tarnished my self-image. I can see now, moreover, how fictional limitations can take on an air of reality. The less I did, the less I felt capable of doing.

It's been quite some time now since I've behaved in such self-centered and self-destructive ways. I've been tempted on occasion, to be sure, but I haven't followed through.

THOUGHT FOR TODAY

Through every action and every thought,
I will stay on the path of wellness.

September 8

"He that strives not to stem his anger's tide,
Does a wild horse without a bridle ride."

COLLEY CIBBER

We do get angry; it would be dishonest and foolish to deny it. Illness and pain sometimes bring out the worst in us. We curse the doctors who can't cure us, fault the government for misspending tax dollars, and shake our fists at God for allowing this to happen to us in the first place.

All too often, we vent our feelings on the friends and family members who share our pain and would give anything to see us well again. We hurt them with our angry outbursts, then lash out again when they well-meaningly assure us that "things could be worse."

When the emotional storm has passed, we feel guilty and unsure of what to do. What *can* we do?

As a start, we shouldn't let too much time go by before apologizing and explaining our true feelings. Later, we can better understand and deal with our anger by looking for underlying causes—frustration or fear, for example. Such self-awareness can go a long way toward defusing anger's explosive potential.

Finally, we should try to remember that misdirected or unresolved anger can never be a force for healing, but more likely will take us in the opposite direction.

THOUGHT FOR TODAY

Besides myself, who else is my anger hurting?

"A bodily disease, which we look upon as whole
and entire within itself, may, after all, be but a
symptom of some ailment in the spiritual part."

NATHANIEL HAWTHORNE

A few years ago a member of my family said to me, not unkindly, "Don't you find it interesting that a person who used to loathe himself as much as you did ended up with cancer and heart disease? And lupus, too, where your immune system attacks your own body?"

I hesitated before responding. The issue is certainly a highly personal one, and I had been caught off guard by his forthrightness. I finally told him, in effect, that it's really up to each person to decide for himself or herself whether emotional factors or past behavior contributed to an illness.

Based on my own life experience, I've not doubted for a moment that the mind and body are interconnected. My physical health always has been affected to some extent by my mental and emotional states.

The fact remains, however, that my illnesses are *present–day* realities. So I therefore choose to invest most of my energy in the physical, emotional, and mental steps that can be taken today, and each new day, to promote healing and wholeness.

THOUGHT FOR TODAY

I can't undo past emotional injury,
but I can practice healthy self-love today.

September 10

> "Renew thyself completely each day;
> do it again, and again, and forever again."
>
> CHINESE PROVERB

Did my emotions and behavior in the past bring about my illnesses? Am I to blame? Does it even matter?

In support groups for lupus and cancer, I've known some people who have been empowered by their belief that negative emotions and self-destructive behavior played a role in causing or exacerbating an illness. I've also had discussions with other people who don't dispute that idea, but would rather focus on today's challenges than explore and analyze the past.

If a person believes that past issues, emotions, and behavior are relevant to a present illness—and, based on that belief, tries to make changes, which might enhance the healing process—it is likely that he or she will benefit. However, the decision is a uniquely personal one. For that reason, such a course of action should not be *imposed* by someone else—neither a relative, close friend, physician, or therapist.

From personal experience, I know that this sort of self-discovery endeavor—in which we search out and try to change underlying emotional patterns—can be helpful only if carried out in nonjudgmental, compassionate, and self-accepting (rather than self-condemning) ways.

THOUGHT FOR TODAY

Exploration of the past is still an option,
but self-blame is not.

"All government, indeed every human benefit and
enjoyment, every virtue, and every prudent act,
is founded on compromise and barter."

EDMUND BURKE

When a medical crisis occurs, family roles change quickly and automatically, but not necessarily smoothly or to the best advantage of all. Indeed, unless role changes are discussed and agreed-to by all concerned, confusion, guilt, resentment, and serious disruption can result.

What are the physical and emotional needs of the father or mother who is suddenly unable to work? What additional responsibilities is the healthy spouse willing and able to handle? Where does the pre-teen daughter fit in? Who will help her balance school, new responsibilities at home, and the normal difficulties of adolescence?

Just because mother, father, and daughter live together doesn't mean each one is intuitively aware of, or fully understands, the others' feelings, needs, and capabilities. Now is the time for everyone to communicate openly and honestly. Now is the time to decide, *together*, what role changes need to be made, and how those changes can work in everyone's best interest.

If roadblocks are encountered, family counseling or a support group can help smooth the way. By finding solutions together, it's likely that the family will become closer than ever before.

THOUGHT FOR TODAY

Work it out; don't fight it out.

September 12

> "One ship drives east and another drives west
> With the selfsame winds that blow.
> 'Tis the set of sails and not the gales
> Which tells us the way to go."
>
> ELLA WHEELER WILCOX

We look around and compare ourselves with others. We decide, "That person is tall; I'm too short." We think, "She's so pretty and I'm so plain." We look, we compare, we judge ourselves harshly, and then we suffer. When we compare our "outsides" with those of others, don't we always end up wanting and feeling inferior?

In truth, as physical beings we are all essentially the same. We are more alike than we are dissimilar, for we all come from the same Source.

Yet we each sense that we are in fact different from anyone else. That difference can of course be found on the inside. It derives from such character traits as self-awareness, positive attitudes, and accurate perspective, which shape our ability to live comfortably and productively.

If we are self-aware, we tend to be honest and courageous, with no need for denial, delusion, or deceit. If we cultivate positive attitudes and work to transform negative ones, we are able to enjoy and appreciate each new day. If we see ourselves right-sized and in proper perspective, then we are better able to reason clearly, coexist harmoniously with our fellows, and live successfully.

THOUGHT FOR TODAY

The important differences are on the inside.

> "The boughs of no two trees have the same arrangement. Nature always produces *individuals;* She never produces classes."
>
> LYDIA MARIA CHILD

You get up the courage to ask the doctor about survival statistics and he's reluctant to get into it. You press him, so he spells out the numbers. You had to know, but now you're sorry you asked.

Intellectually, we understand that statistics are only numbers, yet emotionally we almost always take them personally and interpret them negatively. That's why, when we ask for that sort of information, we need to remind ourselves that statistics are based on averages, and there is no such thing as an average patient.

We should remember, too, that survival statistics can be compromised by such variables as region; physicians' training, knowledge, and experience; and, perhaps most important, by medical advances achieved since the statistics were originally compiled.

That being the case, statistics should be used primarily as a tool to help the healthcare team (of which the patient is a vital member!) decide what treatment course to take. We should try to view statistics objectively and realistically, within the broader context of desire, belief, hope, and faith in God's divine plan for our ultimate good.

THOUGHT FOR TODAY

There is nothing average about me.

September 14

"You may talk of all subjects save one,
namely, your maladies."

RALPH WALDO EMERSON

When people visit us in the hospital, or later, at home, conversations often revolve around the weather, sports, or personalities in the news. Little is said about our illness, and there is no real give and take about what is happening to us and how we are actually feeling. Even when we've known the visitors since childhood, the dialogue tends to be stilted or limited to such superficial exchanges as, "How are you doing?" "Not bad."

The thing is, we *need* to talk about the illness, and so do the people who care for us. This is especially true when there have been changes in our condition, treatment, or prognosis.

When we don't talk about real things (and what is more real than the illness?) we end up feeling lonely, misunderstood and alienated; and we are likely to become annoyed, angry, and ultimately resentful.

So whatever our relationship to the illness—patient, caregiver, or dear friend—we ought to give some thought to how we can best talk about it, what we can say about it, and how we can help others become more comfortable with the subject.

THOUGHT FOR TODAY

Am I willing to take on the illness verbally
as well as medically?

"Travel and change of place impart
new vigor to the mind."
SENECA

As a person who has been challenged by illness for quite a few years, I've tried to develop strategies and techniques that allow me to live comfortably and productively within my physical limitations. At home and around my community I usually apply what I've learned, and I do fairly well. But when I travel it can be quite another story. Sometimes pride, adrenaline, and an overactive sense of adventure take over; I push myself and end up exhausted and in pain.

Here are some of the lessons I'll try to remember next time I travel:

Careful planning, as far in advance as possible, is essential for a successful trip. Since I can't see and do everything, thorough research will help me to make the best choices.

Timing is also crucial. For example, by traveling off-season when possible and by visiting popular attractions midweek rather than on weekends, I can avoid crowds, reduce stress, and get better service.

There are also ways to make airport experiences less frustrating and tiring. I can check luggage instead of lugging it. I can use a courtesy tram or a wheelchair, and I can board the plane early.

THOUGHT FOR TODAY

For my next trip, I'll put common sense
at the top of my packing list.

September 16

"Never argue;
repeat your assertion."
ROBERT OWEN

It's hard to put into words the frustration and humiliation we experience during visits to certain doctors. We feel that we've just passed through enemy territory.

When we pinpoint exactly what takes place in the course of such visits, it's easy to see why we get so upset. We're almost always kept waiting, sometimes for an hour or longer. The doctor seems terribly rushed; he tenses up and appears annoyed when we ask questions. When he does answer, the response is usually cryptic or vague, and we are left wondering what he actually said.

What can we do to solve this problem? To begin with, we can become assertive patients *by speaking up*. We can show the doctor that we are important members of the medical team, capable not only of complying with advice, but also of taking charge of the illness. We can encourage more thorough and satisfying discussions by bringing along a list of symptoms, questions, and comments.

When we are mistreated or made to wait unreasonably, we should complain. The doctor and staff may all be busy professionals, but they are there to serve us. If conditions don't improve after several complaints and discussions, perhaps it's time to move on.

THOUGHT FOR TODAY
I deserve to be treated with consideration and respect.

"If all our misfortunes were laid in one common heap,
whence everyone must take an equal portion, most
people would be content to take their own and depart."
SOCRATES

For a while there, you were feeling really good about yourself and your ability to handle all the medical trauma. When the insurance company denied coverage for the second round of treatment, you knew just what to do and they eventually reversed themselves.

Then, just as you were settling into a routine, a washing machine began to leak, and you found a dead mouse in your clothes closet. Those annoyances almost brought you to your knees.

There seems to be a pattern here. You get through the big stuff just fine, but all too often the minor problems and inconveniences put you over the edge. Had enough? The next time you find yourself close to tears over a broken shoelace, consider these alternatives:

The moment you feel yourself "losing it," stop what you are doing, focus on your breathing, and follow through with whatever serenity-inducing activity works best for you—prayer, meditation, a mantra, reading.

If something can actually be fixed, get it taken care of as soon as you regain your composure. Don't let it drag on and drag you down.

Remember that real friends are not there just for the big things, and that "Let go and let God" can be applied to any circumstance.

THOUGHT FOR TODAY

Put it in perspective.

September 18

"Pray you now,
forget and forgive."

WILLIAM SHAKESPEARE

There may not yet be a cure, but there is always healing. As we now understand it, healing reaches far beyond the physical self and involves our intellect, emotions, and inner spirit.

Along these lines, we have come to realize that the healing process can be severely inhibited by anger, resentment, and hatred. When we harbor these corrosive emotions, we suffer not only soul-sickness but also by intensified physical symptoms.

That is why we practice forgiveness. When we forgive someone we move into the present and out of the past. Forgiveness removes our bitterness while bringing on a new state of consciousness that allows us to coexist peacefully with our fellows.

Sometimes, it is more difficult to forgive ourselves as willingly and completely as we forgive others. The truth is, many of us remain angry at ourselves, holding fast to guilt-provoking memories of past behavior.

Self-forgiveness helps us to acknowledge that we are far different today than we were in the past; that at the time we did the best we could with what we had; and that regardless of our attitudes and actions, God has never stopped loving us unconditionally.

THOUGHT FOR TODAY

And now, to further the healing process,
I will focus on self-forgiveness.

"With the past, I have nothing to do;
nor with the future. I live now."

RALPH WALDO EMERSON

I have been taught to treasure the here and now. Like most people, I often slip back into the past or race forward into the future, but in recent years I've become increasingly successful at living in the now.

I suppose it will always be a challenge to remain in the present moment, especially when pain strikes unexpectedly and then lingers, when a fever spikes abruptly, or when sleep eludes me.

Time becomes distorted when my illness flares out of control. Time loses definition and distinction. Then, it seems that I am living in a separate reality, detached from regular people going about their business, keeping schedules, enjoying each other.

Some mornings, when somnolence gradually gives way to wakefulness and my cool skin tells me that the fever has broken, I drift through time and space. For a while (a minute, an hour, who can tell?) it's unclear where I am or whether it's dawn or dusk.

I know better than to try and fight my way out of such time warps. I do my best to accept them as one more mysterious facet of chronic illness. Eventually I return to true reality, and again embrace the present moment.

THOUGHT FOR TODAY

I may be gone for a while,
but I'll be back.

September 20

"Intuition is the clear conception
of the whole at once."

JOHANN KASPAR LAVATER

Intuition is the inner wisdom that guides us without the aid of intellect or other rational processes. It is the voice within that cautions us to hold back, or urges us to go forward. It admonishes and encourages us, sometimes in a nudging whisper and at other times with fierce insistence.

Now more than ever it is in our best interest to respect and heed intuitive feelings. After all, no one knows our bodies better than we do. By accurately tuning in to physical and emotional messages, and even nuances, our intuition can help us make wise choices and sound decisions concerning our health.

For example, intuition can override an adventurous nature and let us know when to use discretion. Intuition can help us determine what we can handle and what we can not, when to ask for help and when to push ourselves.

Our intuitive voice can also alert us to subtle new symptoms, and can help us know when to take action and when to "wait and see." For all of these reasons, our goal is to listen carefully and develop ever-greater trust in our caring and protective inner voice.

THOUGHT FOR TODAY

I will not let the clamorous voices of fear, ego, and self-will drown out my intuition.

> "Health and good estate of body are above all gold,
> and a strong body above infinite wealth."
>
> APOCRYPHA, ECCLESIASTICUS 30:15

The worst part of visiting my accountant each spring is the time we spend adding up medical expenses. I read off the seemingly endless totals for each doctor, lab, pharmacy, and hospital, while the accountant's fingers click away on the calculator keys. Finally, he looks up, tells me the total, and shakes his head sympathetically. And I always respond in pretty much the same way: "I could have taken my whole family around the world with that kind of money!"

Obviously, I've been troubled with recurring feelings of guilt and anger about money spent on my illnesses—money that could "serve far better purposes." I suffer through the inner turmoil until it occurs to me, one more time, that *there is no better purpose.* If I'm not well, how can I enjoy a new bicycle, new power tools, a new car? If I'm not well, how can I travel around the block, let alone around the world?

Each year I put myself through the emotional guilt wringer. I end up asking myself the same basic question, and then come up with the same reassuring answer: What better purpose for money than healing and wellness? The money may be gone, but I'm not.

THOUGHT FOR TODAY

When I am able to put a dollar value
on health and life, then I will be able
to say how much is "too much."

> "It is well to live that
> one may learn."
>
> MIGUEL DE CERVANTES SAAVEDRA

Anyone who has ever been gravely ill is familiar with the profound insights we can gain from such an experience. It becomes clear, quickly and dramatically, that we are entirely mortal, that life is a gift to be treasured, and that each precious day ought to be lived as fully and joyously as possible.

That is the "big" revelation, the one we share with friends, family, and co-workers, and they know exactly what we are talking about. But illness can bring other important insights as well. As we gradually recover, whether by active rehabilitation or bed rest, we can gain deep awarenesses about other aspects of our lives.

We may come to realize, for example, that certain relationships are toxic and beyond repair, or that others deserve reconstruction. We may see that our practice of moving from house to house and city to city is an always unsuccessful maneuver to escape our own unresolved inner conflicts. We may discover that our harsh treatment of others is a reflexive extension of negative feelings we have about ourselves.

When these insights come, we should be open to them. We can learn from them, grow because of them, and use them as catalysts to improve our quality of life.

THOUGHT FOR TODAY

Illness can teach. Am I willing to learn?

"Fear of danger is ten thousand times
more terrifying than danger itself."

DANIEL DEFOE

It seems like a million years ago, but there was a time, before this illness was finally diagnosed, when you were reluctant to find out what it was. You even tried to hide your symptoms from family members to forestall being pressured into seeking medical advice. It's so very clear now that fear and fear alone was behind your avoidance, motivating every decision and action.

Many new fears have arisen since then, and you've gradually learned how to understand them, deal with them and, if need be, live with them. When a new fear surfaces these days, you think back to that overwhelming pre-diagnosis fear and how you found the courage to overcome it. That same courage, you affirm, can see you through just about anything.

When you face an unfamiliar challenge and the knot in your stomach tells you that you are becoming afraid, you try to remember these powerful and unchanging realities: Fear can be replaced with faith, the deep-down conviction that God is always at your side to protect and care for you. No fear is too large, too small, or too irrational for God's concern and involvement.

THOUGHT FOR TODAY

Fear distorts reality. Faith dissolves fear.

> "God helps those
> who help themselves."
>
> BENJAMIN FRANKLIN

I'm hardly a stranger to pain and most of the time, thankfully, I'm able to manage or at least live with it. Recently, however, I suffered through an episode which seemed to dwarf anything I had previously known. It involved bone loss, nerve extraction, and other dental horrors. Pain-killers did little to relieve my agony.

The experience turned my life upside down. For two weeks I couldn't eat properly, sleep soundly, or think clearly. When I finally recovered I had lost much of my self-confidence, and had begun to rely on my wife to help me make even the simplest decisions.

When things settled down, she reminded me that I had gone through similar episodes of insecurity and self-doubt in the past following other surgeries and severe lupus flare-ups. My wife further reminded me (*reassured* me, actually) that I am strong, capable, and dependable.

It was an important learning experience for me. I can see clearly now that I must take action following episodes of prolonged discomfort or acute pain. It's essential to build myself up mentally and emotionally, by affirming, with deep conviction, "I am strong, I am capable, I am dependable."

THOUGHT FOR TODAY

I will not let pain diminish me in any way.

"Do not spoil what you have by desiring what
you have not: remember that what you now have
was once among the things you only hoped for."

EPICURUS

A friend of mine with breast cancer began a course of radiation and chemotherapy. During the second month, she experienced debilitating fatigue and nausea. As a result, she had to spend much of her time resting.

My friend phoned one evening. "I have a small aquarium with just one fish, a beautiful blue and red Betta," she said. "I spent the longest time today just watching him swim round and round his bowl, through the little plastic plants, so slowly and so gracefully."

"I'd never paid that much attention to him," she continued, "and it suddenly dawned on me what a blessing it is to be quiet and serene, to feel content and complete in the moment. And I thought, everything I have, I have right now. That's all I really want, and that's all I really need. That's all there really *is*.

"Then," my friend said, "I thought back to all the running around I used to do, and it seemed so ridiculous. Always in a rush, always worried about what I was going to do next, instead of living in the moment. I can't think of one good reason to ever want to go back to that kind of life."

THOUGHT FOR TODAY

I will live this moment, this most
precious moment, to the fullest.

September 26

> "Faith is like a lily,
> lifted high and white."

CHRISTINA ROSSETTI

The door to the hospital chapel is ajar and you can see a lone woman kneeling in prayer. You would like to do the same, to ask for God's help, but the whole idea of religion is somehow intimidating.

Many of us have had similar reservations. We wanted to seek spiritual solutions, to find comfort, guidance, and possibly even healing grace in a Power greater than ourselves—but we were unwilling to embrace a religious creed or doctrine. Because we confused spirituality with religion, the power of faith seemed remote and inaccessible.

We have since developed a new belief system, each of us in our own way. While some have been able to find spiritual faith through organized religion, others have found a God of their own understanding. This approach provides the personal freedom and flexibility we needed to develop a faith that works.

Spirituality is as much a way of living as it is a way of believing. By practicing such spiritual principles as tolerance, forgiveness, kindness, and acceptance, we have been uplifted. Through faith and trust in a Higher Power, we no longer have to depend solely on our own limited resources when meeting life's challenges.

THOUGHT FOR TODAY

God is everywhere, available to everyone.

"We are responsible for the effort not the outcome."
ANONYMOUS

At the beginning, following the diagnosis and initial treatment, we were of course bewildered and frightened. When the healthcare team and our family took over, we were not only grateful but enormously relieved.

Even later, when the treatment schedule was familiar and our days became more predictable, we continued to rely completely on our doctors, nurses, and loved ones. They were quite willing to remain in charge, to care for us, and to try as best they could to move us along the path to wellness.

Eventually, however, we learned a challenging lesson: No matter how much others want to help and can help us to heal, the ultimate responsibility is ours, and the basic effort must come from us. Physicians prescribe treatment regimens, but it's up to us to implement them. Rehabilitation specialists teach beneficial exercises, but we alone can follow through. Nutritionists recommend what to eat or avoid, but at the table we're the ones who bring the food to our mouths.

In the final analysis, then, we are responsible—for learning all we can about our illness, for developing positive attitudes, for listening carefully to our bodies, and for nurturing hope.

THOUGHT FOR TODAY

Thanks for being there when I needed you, and for remaining at my side. From now on, though, it's mostly up to me.

> "Life's a tumble-about thing
> of ups and downs."
>
> BENJAMIN DISRAELI

I wake up on certain mornings feeling remarkably well, and my mind races with joyful expectations of all the things I'll be able to do during the day. But then, within a few hours, everything changes. Joints stiffen, pain rises, and fatigue overwhelms me. I am devastated.

One of the infuriating things about chronic illness is the uncertainty of it all. It's almost impossible to know, day to day or even hour to hour, how I'm going to be feeling and what I'm going to be capable of doing.

In many ways, living with chronic illness is like riding a roller coaster. There are slow and smooth ascensions, precipitous plunges, occasional level spots, and always nerve-jangling unpredictability. However, I've learned that just because I'm on a physical roller coaster, that doesn't mean I have to take my emotions along for the ride. It doesn't mean I have to swing from elation to devastation and back again with every twist, turn, rise or fall of my illnesses.

That's the challenge today and every day: to keep my emotions steady, stable, and level no matter how I'm feeling physically.

THOUGHT FOR TODAY
_____
Unrealistic expectations are a recipe for emotional pain.

"The only conquests, which are permanent and leave no regrets, are our conquests over ourselves."

NAPOLEON BONAPARTE

How can we resist the wave of regret that sometimes sweeps us off the path of wellness? What can we do to counteract those destructive thoughts that tell us *we* were responsible for our illness, or that we wasted years of good health?

There is much we can do to anchor ourselves in reality. To begin with, we can try to recognize that such perceptions of the past are almost always distorted and exaggerated. Yes, we worked hard and played hard. But those years were wonderful, and wouldn't we make those same choices again? Maybe we didn't realize all of our dreams, but our lives certainly have been rich and meaningful.

Some people find it useful to write about their regrets, or simply to discuss them with a close friend. By bringing regretful thoughts of the past into the open, we can drain them of their power and regain an accurate perspective.

Finally, we can do our utmost to forgive ourselves for mistakes we actually did make. We can remind ourselves that at the time we did the best we could with what we had. And we can surrender, asking for God's help in letting go of the past.

THOUGHT FOR TODAY

Feelings of regret may arise from time to time, but I need not give them power.

> "A man's first care should be to avoid
> the reproaches of his own heart."
>
> JOSEPH ADDISON

Every one of us is sometimes dragged down emotionally by an illness, way down. We then become vulnerable to old ideas and distorted views of the past. We may become regretful, castigating ourselves for doing too much for too long, for using up our energy stores, for burning ourselves out. At that point, we can easily become convinced that we're to blame for the illness.

Or we may be overwhelmed with another form of regret, berating ourselves for risks never taken, adventures never experienced, dreams never realized—for all the years of "good health wasted."

For me, those occasional dark-of-the-night regrets revolve around self-centered excess. Too much alcohol; too many cigarettes; too much junk food; not enough exercise; decades of physical and emotional self-destructiveness.

No matter what the nature of our regrets, we're learning that nothing could be more counterproductive to wellness and peace of mind. Guilt for past actions or inactions makes us feel unworthy and undeserving. Invariably, such a burden of self-blame prevents us from doing our very best to recover.

THOUGHT FOR TODAY

There's a cure for self-blame.
It's called self-acceptance.

October

October 1

> "Pain is deeper than all thought;
> laughter is higher than all pain."
>
> ELBERT HUBBARD

I'll never forget the first alcoholism support-group meeting I attended. Sick, shaky, and miserable, the last thing I expected that night was to be laughing uncontrollably. But that's exactly what did happen when the speaker told a bizarre, tasteless, and self-deprecating joke about a drunk who had been run over by a train. It was my first experience with the healing power of laughter.

Humor can have a therapeutic effect on any number of illnesses. It's been proven that laughter relieves stress and may thereby strengthen the immune system. The late Norman Cousins, who studied this phenomenon for many years, summed it up by commenting that laughter can be a significant part of recovery and is part of the full range of positive human emotions as is love, faith, hope, determination, and purpose.

From my own perspective, I know that when I laugh I feel good; when I laugh I take deep, relaxing breaths; when I laugh my mind is cleared of negative thoughts and feelings; when I laugh I reinforce my conviction that life is a gift to be treasured.

THOUGHT FOR TODAY

Not only in the best of times, but also in the worst of times, I will seek moments of lightness.

"...I would that thus, when I shall see The hour of death
draw near to me, Hope, blossoming within my heart,
May look to heaven as I depart."

WILLIAM CULLEN BRYANT

When people who are terminally ill know that death is imminent, they and those close to them usually take steps to put their affairs in order. Wills are drawn up or revised, funeral wishes are expressed, personal mementoes are passed along. Such actions can bring about comforting feelings of completion.

But other actions, of a different sort, can result in a more meaningful sense of closure. By moving beyond material concerns and focusing on relationships—by communicating intimate thoughts and messages long held back—the person who is ill, as well as family members and friends, can experience a true sense of inner peace.

Perhaps there is an amends to be made or forgiveness to be offered. Perhaps the time has arrived for a hidden secret to be brought to light. Unanswered questions can be resolved, explanations can at long last be given.

For everyone involved this is the perfect time, if ever there was one, to clearly express feelings that may not have been fully expressed in the past. Feelings of kinship and respect; feelings of pride and approval; feelings of love.

THOUGHT FOR TODAY

I will be loving and open;
I will be courageous.

> "To overcome difficulties is to experience
> the full delight of existence."
>
> ARTHUR SCHOPENHAUER

Somewhere back in time, when the pills had stopped working and the doctors were considering a nerve block, you remember someone saying with deep conviction, "You can learn a great deal from pain."

That prophecy (perhaps it was only a suggestion) turned out to hold an abundance of truth. You have indeed learned a lot from pain, and the knowledge you've gained has made your days and nights tolerable and even enjoyable again. These are some of the most valuable lessons:

You have learned how to change your attitudes and reactions toward pain, thereby enhancing your ability to manage it and limit its influence on your life. You now know, for example, that to struggle against pain only causes tension and even more pain, and that pain tends to diminish when you try to accept it calmly.

The advent of chronic pain does not doom you to the role of victim; you need not suffer perennially and passively. Your tolerance for pain is now greater than you could have imagined. And you are a lot stronger and far more resourceful than you thought.

THOUGHT FOR TODAY

Pain ebbs and flows, changing moment
by moment and second by second.
It is changing right now.

"Every day, in every way,
I am getting better and better."
ÉMILE COUÉ

My cousin had a heart attack not long ago. When I called to cheer him up, we began to compare notes. I told him about lifestyle changes I had gradually made following my heart surgery, and all he talked about was his new diet and the no-fat recipes he and his wife had been preparing. He proudly described a new electronic scale that weighed out portions by the gram.

Later, I remembered that I too had been zealous about my diet during the initial recuperation period. I soon learned that diet is but one factor in the wellness equation. It has become just as important to pay serious attention to all areas of life that influence my health and sense of well-being, including exercise, rest, stress reduction, and the elimination of such negative attitudes as judgmentalism and cynicism. Each of these activities is valuable in and of itself; all of them, working together, inspire hope and optimism in my life.

I tried to describe the broad focus of my wellness activities to my cousin, but I'm not sure he really heard me. Perhaps that's just as well. It's something he's better off learning on his own.

THOUGHT FOR TODAY

The more I do for myself,
the better I feel about myself.

"The highest compact we can make with our fellow is,
'Let there be truth between us two for evermore.'"

RALPH WALDO EMERSON

Honest and open communication is a vital ingredient in any relationship. We all know that. And it's even more essential when one of the partners is seriously ill. There are times, though, when we may be tempted to withhold the truth from a loved one.

Let's say that our most recent medical test results are less than encouraging. The doctor confirms that we've taken a turn for the worse, and recommends more aggressive treatment. Now we're not sure how to handle it. On the one hand we want to tell our spouse the whole truth; on the other, we want to hold back and spare him or her further emotional pain.

Holding back facts about an illness is rarely a good idea, no matter how noble our intentions. A loved one has to know the whole truth in order to adjust emotionally and be understanding and supportive in the best possible way. Moreover, there is always a price to pay for dishonesty, whether by commission or omission. By causing emotional pressure, dishonesty can adversely affect the healing process.

Granted, it takes courage to put new and unwelcome facts on the table. But at such times honesty is the kindest and most loving action we can take.

THOUGHT FOR TODAY

If the tables were turned, wouldn't I
want to know the whole truth?

"Tell me and I'll forget, show me and I may remember;
involve me and I'll understand."

CHINESE PROVERB

Radiology, hematology, nuclear medicine. EKG, MRI, CAT Scan. Tests, tests, and more tests. The needles, clamps, and probes are awful enough, but there's also the unpleasant preparation—the laxatives, the fasting, the shaving. But the very worst part, the part that upsets you most, is not knowing what the tests are for, what the costs will be, and what the results will mean.

What can you do to cut through the confusion and frustration, to overcome some of the stress, and possibly reduce the expense? Most importantly, you can ask questions. As soon as a test is prescribed, ask your doctor questions such as these:

Why are you recommending this test? Can you talk me through the procedure step by step? How long will it take? What about side effects? How much will it cost? Will the results be clear-cut? Do I really need this test, or are there less costly alternatives?

If you ask these and other relevant questions, and insist on understandable answers, you'll be surprised at how your confusion and anxiety will lessen. And you'll be thrilled at how your sense of control will increase.

THOUGHT FOR TODAY

I have a right to know.

October 7

> "There is no vulture like despair."
>
> GEORGE GRANVILLE

Every once in a while I allow myself to become angry, disgusted, and completely fed up with being sick. I growl and curse and sometimes even lash out. Then, after the rush of negativity has ebbed, I wonder dejectedly, "*Now* what?"

If I permit myself to remain fed up I'll sink even lower on the emotional scale. If, on the other hand, I choose to find my way back to the acceptance of illness and its daily challenges, I can salve my self-inflicted wounds and salvage the day.

When I choose a positive response—the path of acceptance—to "Now what?" there are actions that have worked for me in the past. I talk to a friend, in person or on the phone, honestly admitting how my self-pity has dragged me down. I try to talk also about some of the good things in my life, the blessings.

At some point I turn to God, surrendering my will and asking Him to help me accept the things I can't change. Finally, I try to do something nice for someone else. For me, that's the best way to get over feeling disgusted and fed up.

THOUGHT FOR TODAY

Feeling fed up is a dubious luxury
I really can't afford.

"All prayers are answered if we are willing to
admit that sometimes the answer is 'no.'"
ANONYMOUS

We want to help ourselves heal, Lord knows we do. Through strenuous effort we want somehow to relieve our pain, assuage our fear, smooth away the rough spots, and find solutions. With every fiber of our being, we want to restore and uplift ourselves, to once again experience joy and peace of mind.

Yet the harder we try, the greater our frustration and sense of failure. At times like this it seems that there is almost nothing we can do to help ourselves. We feel utterly powerless.

But there is power in prayer. Through prayer we can renew our partnership with God. Silently, unobtrusively, yet powerfully, His grace can achieve what is beyond human capability. When we acknowledge and affirm that reality, we open a channel for His healing spirit to shine through.

We want to help ourselves and now we have found a very special way to do so. By turning to God we can bring grace and serenity back to our lives. We can place our trust in God and find great comfort in His divine plan for our ultimate well-being.

THOUGHT FOR TODAY

I acknowledge my own powerlessness;
I affirm the power of God.

October 9

> "The art of medicine consists in amusing the
> patient while nature cures the disease."
>
> VOLTAIRE

We have flashbacks to an earlier time. The orthopedic surgeon promises that the saw will cut through only the plaster cast and not our skin; he is certain that our leg will soon be strong and well enough for skiing. The family doctor removes the last gauze pad from our appendectomy incision and smilingly assures us that it is healing quickly.

Now that we are chronically ill, with pain as a constant companion, it's tempting to think of those earlier times as "the good old days." However, we've discovered that such a perspective is not only depressing emotionally, but debilitating physically.

What we've begun to do, instead, is redefine our terms. Where once "healing" meant completion, perfect closure, and a return to physical wholeness, we now see it primarily as an internal process. By healing on the inside we are able to become free of fear, anger, resentment, and guilt in order to make the best of each available moment.

And where "wellness" once meant an absence of illness, it has come to mean the possession of character assets such as selflessness, patience, humility and, above all, acceptance.

THOUGHT FOR TODAY

What I will focus on—what I can achieve—
is healing on the inside.

"An arrow may fly through the air and leave no trace;
but an ill thought leaves a trail like a serpent."

CHARLES MACKAY

For reasons I haven't yet been able to fathom, my mind sometimes tries to get the best of me. Because pain tends to be a point of particular sensitivity and vulnerability, my negative inner dialogue usually goes something like this: *I can't stand it anymore... I look terrible... It's such an effort to do anything... The cancer is back... I'm worthless... Nobody really understands.*

When such thoughts gallop wildly across my consciousness these days, I try quickly to rein them in. Unchecked, they can cause serious harm, debilitating me physically and emotionally.

I've learned over the years that if I hold a thought long enough, it becomes an expectation. For example, if I believe that "nobody really understands," I'm likely to set myself apart from others. If I expect a bad day, that's what I'll create for myself.

As with so many aspects of life, it comes down to personal choices. I can choose and expect alienation or connectedness; I can choose and expect despair or hope.

THOUGHT FOR TODAY

Negative thoughts are not realities,
unless I make them so.

> "Grief drives men into habits of serious reflection,
> sharpens the understanding and softens the heart."
>
> JOHN ADAMS

It comes to us at different times and in different places—in a hospital bed or our own bed at home, during a family outing, or in the darkness of a movie theater. We suddenly realize that illness has drastically changed our lives, and we are overwhelmed with a deep sense of loss.

What has happened is that we have begun to grieve. Although we usually associate grieving with death, the process can follow any major loss. In the case of chronic illness or pain, we experience many losses, some immediately apparent and others less obvious or delayed. We may lose the ability to participate in sports we once enjoyed, or to travel extensively. We may have to put aside certain dreams and aspirations.

For people with chronic illness, grieving is not only normal, but necessary. By working our way through the stages of grief—denial, anger, bargaining, depression, and acceptance—we are able to acknowledge and come to terms with our losses. The grief process allows us to let go of our former lifestyle and goals, in order to take advantage of new opportunities and accept the challenge of building and enjoying a new life.

THOUGHT FOR TODAY
***
By accepting my losses, I have
everything to gain.

"One joy shatters a hundred griefs."

CHINESE PROVERB

Although the stages of grief can be as painful as the illness or injury that brought them on, the process itself is ultimately healing and life-enhancing.

Denial is the first stage. This is when we question the reality of the illness, the need for treatment, and so on. Denial buffers the initial shock, and allows us to collect ourselves.

Anger marks the second stage of the grief process. We rail at life's unfairness; we lash out at others; we shake our fist at God. Anger is a potent and potentially destructive emotion, to be sure, yet if we suppress it we risk becoming walking time bombs. Anger is unavoidable, but there are constructive ways to get through it.

Next comes bargaining. We try to make deals with God. We'll promise almost anything to get our health back.

When we realize the futility of trying to deny or bargain away our illness, depression often sets in. We may be overcome by sadness, unexpected tears, or an inability to function at all. These are powerful emotions, and it takes time to resolve them.

In the final stage of grieving, we achieve acceptance. We put aside despair about our lost selves, and learn to focus instead on the opportunities that lie ahead.

THOUGHT FOR TODAY

I will get through denial, anger, bargaining, and depression. I will achieve acceptance.

October 13

> "Anger sets the house on fire ... it is a short madness, and an eternal enemy to discourse and sober counsels and fair conversation."
>
> JEREMY TAYLOR

Just as we're beginning to come to terms with the seriousness of our illness, and perhaps settling into a relatively productive routine, we become aware of a new problem in our household. There is a lot of anger. Our husband, wife, or partner—the one who is not ill—is short-tempered and irritable much of the time. Periodically, especially when we're feeling poorly and experiencing more pain than usual, their anger is explosive. We are hurt by their outbursts, but try to be understanding. After all, haven't we let them down? Who wouldn't be angry at a loss of companionship, and an increase in financial burdens and household responsibilities? So we walk on eggshells, tiptoe around the anger, and are careful not to complain. But then, one very special evening, we open up to each other and have a heart-to-heart talk. To our great relief, we discover that our partner is not angry at us and never has been. The anger has to do with the illness, with overpowering feelings of frustration and helplessness. Their anger comes from feeling out of control, and sensing that this time love may not be enough.

THOUGHT FOR TODAY

I will try to understand my partner's anger and not take it personally.

"It is a mathematical fact that fifty percent of all doctors graduate in the bottom half of their class."

ANONYMOUS

I can't begin to count the number of doctors' offices, medical clinics, and hospitals I've been to over the past several decades. During a recent visit for blood tests, it occurred to me that a significant change is taking place in such facilities. I'm not talking about technology or treatment approaches but, rather, about the attitudes and behavior of patients like myself.

In the past we tended to go along passively with whatever recommendations our doctors made. We had been conditioned to put medical professionals on an elevated plane; we automatically consented and almost never questioned.

More and more these days, however, we as patients are recognizing and exercising our rights to seek second opinions, to pursue alternatives, to make decisions. Our awareness level has risen, and it's become clear that we must be actively involved in our own health care. After all, we are the ones who are ill, and we are the ones who must do our utmost to become well again. That includes learning all we can about the illness; seeking new options; evaluating the members of our medical team; and, if necessary, creating a new team.

THOUGHT FOR TODAY

Is it time to change my role from bench-sitter to team leader?

October 15

> "Ah me! The Prison House of Pain!—what lessons
> there are bought!—Lessons of a sublimer strain
> than any elsewhere taught."
>
> FLORENCE EARLE COATES

The other morning I accidentally dropped my wife's favorite coffee mug. I remember thinking, as I swept up the fragments, that the day was off to a horrible start, and it would probably get worse. The prophecy was self-fulfilling: By noon I tipped over my own coffee mug and had a full-blown temper tantrum while unsuccessfully trying to fix a broken screen door.

Not until mid-afternoon did I understand the reason for my clumsiness and irritability. My joints had been so inflamed and painful when I woke up that I could hardly get out of bed. No wonder I became impatient and easily rattled while doing even simple tasks.

The pattern is always so clear in retrospect. If only I could sharpen my awareness and make the pain/attitude/behavior connection earlier. That way I would change my expectations and actions during difficult days. I would slow my pace, stay warmer, let someone else do the driving. I would give myself permission to do less, to rest more, to ask for help. And, if I became frustrated, I would remind myself of what was going on and why.

THOUGHT FOR TODAY

I respect pain, and I try to accept pain,
but I will not be controlled by pain.

"What we have to learn to do we learn by doing."

ARISTOTLE

The tests are over, the results are in, and now you're back home. Your family is close at hand, eagerly offering support and advice. Every five minutes, or so it seems, someone is telling you to lie down, move around, eat this, avoid that, quit your job, and on and on.

Because of the newly diagnosed illness, your world has been turned upside down. Your emotions are all over the place. So when loved ones try to assume the decision-making role, you may be inclined to give in and let them.

This usually isn't a good idea. While it's natural for well-intentioned family members to jump in and try to run your household, manage your time, and take control, their efforts will almost certainly lead to hurt feelings and resentment on all sides.

As soon as possible after a diagnosis, it's important to cooperatively establish a set of ground rules. Gently remind family members that you are your own person and that you still know your body better than anyone. Explain that because the illness has taken certain aspects of control away from you, it's crucial to retain control whenever and wherever you can.

THOUGHT FOR TODAY

Good intentions don't always
lead to good results.

> "Obstacles cannot crush me. Every obstacle
> yields to stern resolve. He who is fixed to a
> star does not change his mind."
>
> LEONARDO DA VINCI

When good health was something we took for granted, many of us were highly goal-oriented. We gauged our progress in life (and sometimes even our self-worth) by targets set and met. We had goals in areas ranging from career and financial security to physical and emotional fitness. Some of these goals are still attainable, but others may have had to be modified, put on hold, or dropped entirely.

Sickness or injury notwithstanding, it's still important to have a clear direction. We still want to move forward and experience personal and spiritual growth. That's why we're setting some new goals for ourselves, along these lines:

To become more accepting of our limitations and disabilities. To regain self-assurance and optimism. To become more confident in our ability to transcend pain. To strengthen our relationship with God through regular prayer and meditation. To become less resentful, and more forgiving. To take actions to improve our self-image and develop healthy self-love. To reduce stress and become less anxious, depressed, and angry. To offer support and hope to others similarly afflicted.

THOUGHT FOR TODAY

How can I grow and move forward today?

> "Cherish your yesterdays; dread your tomorrows;
> but live your todays."
>
> ANONYMOUS

How long do I have to live? We all ask this question from time to time, silently or aloud, in sickness and in health. In most cases no one can know the answer.

Despite this reality, some people continue to wonder, sometimes obsessively, "how much time" they have left, and then become terrified of the imagined answer. Needless to say, this mental and emotional process is an exercise in futility. It serves no purpose except to cast a pall over each day and to tarnish the quality of life overall.

No matter what our situation, we can always choose to focus on living rather than dying. We can choose faith over despair and hope over resignation. We can adamantly refuse to be tyrannized by pain, uncertainty, or fear.

We may not be all we wish to be physically, but we do have clear choices concerning our mental, emotional, and spiritual condition. A day at a time, we can exercise these choices by committing ourselves to mental clarity, emotional stability, and spiritual connectedness. In short, we can insist on living each day to its fullest.

THOUGHT FOR TODAY

I will live well, and fully, and gracefully.

October 19

> "Nowhere can man find a quieter or more untroubled retreat than in his own soul."
>
> MARCUS AURELIUS

We've had the feeling for some time now that meditation could be a valuable addition to our treatment program. But we never seem to get it right. In fact, during several tries at meditating we became even more tense than when we had begun.

Recently we've read up on the subject, and also have been given some food for thought in our support group. Perhaps meditation hasn't "worked," it was suggested, because we approached it with goals that were far too specific. We set out to gain wisdom, to become refreshed, to have our pain relieved, or to be quickly calmed down.

Come to think of it, each time we pursued such specific goals and failed to achieve them, we felt disappointed and restless, and then became unwilling to continue meditating.

Could it be that for us the primary purpose of meditation is to simply *let ourselves be,* to quietly and non-judgmentally observe our thoughts and feelings as they flow across our consciousness? If in the healing stillness we then gain wisdom, lose pain, and become refreshed and calm, so much the better.

THOUGHT FOR TODAY

The right way to meditate is the way that works best for me.

"Not only is there but one way of doing things rightly;
there is only one way of seeing them, and that
is seeing the whole of them."

JOHN RUSKIN

I remember waking up one morning not long ago and immediately feeling like hell. When I hobbled into the bathroom and routinely opened the medicine cabinet, I was suddenly dismayed by the array of medications. There were pills, lotions, ointments, and drops for at least seven different ailments and illnesses. I shook my head and said to myself, "There's so much *wrong* with me!"

I carried that thought around for a good part of the day. It weighed heavily and dragged my spirits down. As evening approached, I realized that I had been perceiving myself in that same self-pitying way for quite some time. I had been focusing primarily on the areas of my body that give me trouble, and all the things that are "wrong" with me.

I vowed then to try to shift my perspective, to focus on an overriding reality: There's a lot more *right* with me than there is *wrong* with me. That affirmation, and the effort that followed it, brought me a great sense of relief that night. Hopefully, it will do so in the future as well.

THOUGHT FOR TODAY

What's really wrong is the way
I sometimes see myself.

> "Shame is Pride's cloak."
>
> WILLIAM BLAKE

A friend of mine has an illness that qualifies him for a handicapped parking permit. But he refuses to apply for one. Another friend has received such a permit, but has used it only once. "I parked in a special spot in front of the market and this man shrieked at me, 'You're not sick, you faker!'" she recalled with a shudder.

Like my two friends, many of us with physical challenges are reluctant to use special parking permits for various reasons. If we don't appear ill or disabled "on the outside," we may fear being confronted by ignorant people. We may not be willing to acknowledge that our condition is serious enough to require special treatment. Or we may fear that our use of a special permit or similar consideration will fuel the self-pitying "victim" mentality that sometimes flares within us.

The reality, of course, is that special requirements for an illness need not diminish us in any way—provided that we have the right attitude. When life becomes more complicated and difficult, doesn't it make sense to do everything we can to ease the burden?

THOUGHT FOR TODAY

I won't let self-consciousness, embarrassment— or pride—influence my healthcare decisions.

> "As long as you live,
> keep learning how to live."
>
> SENECA

If you were to look back through your personal history, it's likely that certain events would stand out. You'd remember most vividly the truly transitional experiences, the ones that dramatically changed the course of your life. Marriage, the birth of a child, a career change, the death of a loved one, divorce—these are but several examples of life-altering events.

Now that you have a chronic illness, your life has again begun to change in ways you couldn't have imagined. At present, it may seem that the illness has forced you on a detour, in a direction not only unforeseen but also unacceptable. However, as time goes on and the path becomes more clearly marked, your unplanned journey could well become rich and rewarding.

If you embrace life-enhancing principles, you will experience new levels of awareness and come to know yourself better than ever before. You will develop greater self-confidence and self-respect. You will reclaim a sense of wonder and reverence for life, and become grateful for each new day. You will learn to choose hope over despair, acceptance over anger, and faith over fear.

THOUGHT FOR TODAY

With God's help, you can find tools
to transcend pain and illness.

October 23

"In time of sickness the
soul collects itself anew."

PROVERB

We unhesitatingly take every possible action to rid ourselves of the physical causes of illness, no matter what toxic form they take—bacterial, viral, or parasitical. We utilize every available therapy to strengthen our immune system, stabilize our blood pressure, and lower our sedimentation rate.

But what about soul sickness? Isn't it just as important to become free of toxins that can't be revealed by blood tests and X-rays? The fact is that certain negative emotions—resentment, remorse, and recrimination, in particular—can be just as deadly as any virus or cell gone awry.

Nothing contaminates us more than a long-held, festering grudge. Nothing requires a heavier emotional investment than our endless rehearsals of acts of retribution.

Whether we are healthy, ill, or on the road to recovery, none of us can afford to squander precious energies on ghosts of the past, or phantoms of the present and future. We need to reserve all of our inner strength for constructive purposes, for goals that actually can be achieved. Therefore, even as we diligently follow procedures to heal our bodies, so too must we do everything possible to purify our souls.

THOUGHT FOR TODAY

Are toxic emotions hindering my recovery?

"No child of God sins to that degree as to make himself incapable of forgiveness."

JOHN BUNYAN

Do we want to remain contaminated by resentment and other poisonous emotions? Must we continually probe and re-infect our psychic wounds? Or are we now ready, finally, to be healed?

The soul-sickness of resentment can best be overcome with forgiveness. When we forgive someone, the only thing we give up is our own pain, no matter how grievous the real or imagined wrongs committed against us.

But that is not all. Forgiveness quenches the fires of pain that have been smoldering within us, perhaps for years. Forgiveness makes it possible to save and rebuild once-precious relationships. Forgiveness helps us to grow spiritually by enabling us, once again, to be understanding, compassionate, and accepting.

If it is difficult for us to forgive there are ways to make it easier. We can empathetically try to place ourselves in the shoes of those we need to forgive, thereby gaining insight into their personal backgrounds, influences, and motivations. We can acknowledge that we also are capable of wrongdoing and may someday wish to be forgiven. And we can ask God to help us become *entirely willing* to forgive, so that the healing process may begin.

THOUGHT FOR TODAY

Forgiveness heals.

> "I pray thee, O God,
> that I may be beautiful within."
>
> SOCRATES

More times than you can count, people have urged you over the last several months to "think positively." That makes all the sense in the world, to be sure, and you always respond with a vigorous nod and a cheery, "Oh, I will!"

But how exactly does one think positively? It's not as if you can throw a switch and instantaneously change your mindset and outlook. Positive thinking requires not only desire, but conscious effort on a daily basis. Here are some suggestions to help you transform your thinking:

- Reflect on past successes you've had with projects or career goals, for example, as well as with relationships, decision-making, and personal challenges.

- Instead of focusing on all the things that are "wrong" with you at present, look carefully at all that is right. Concentrate on the activities you enjoy instead of those now beyond your reach; be grateful for your capabilities.

- Look for, think about, and point out the good in people, places, and situations. And if you have to mentally project into the future, try to do so with hope, faith, and positive expectations rather than with despair, fear, and pessimism.

THOUGHT FOR TODAY

I can change my mind—*literally.*

"Pain forces even
the innocent to lie."

PUBLILIUS SYRUS

When the pain struck in the middle of the night I knew exactly where it was, what it was, and how it felt. I knew it so well I could have written lyrics about it.

The next morning in the doctor's office I was anything but lyrical. In fact, I hardly discussed the pain at all and directed the doctor's attention to other matters. Then, on the way home, I felt like a fool. If the doctor doesn't have a complete picture of my symptoms, how can he properly treat me?

Later, I asked myself why I had been so "heroic." Perhaps I hadn't wanted to add to the doctor's burdens; after all, he deals with people's pain all day long, and what a drag that must be. Or perhaps I wanted his approval and felt I would be more likely to get it if I didn't complain.

That thought reminded me of what it was like growing up. In my family we never admitted we were in pain, let alone complained about it. We were taught to grin and bear it. And that's why, to this day, I sometimes try to show that I am strong, that I can handle it.

THOUGHT FOR TODAY

Hiding the pain hinders the healing.

October 27

"Apprehension, uncertainty, waiting, expectation, fear of surprise, do a patient more harm than any exertion."
FLORENCE NIGHTINGALE

At the end of the consultation the oncologist takes our arm and says softly, "We'll do everything we can. But there are no guarantees." In that moment, every test result and every encouraging word is suddenly overshadowed by stark uncertainty. So many unanswered questions, so many fears! How does one cope?

Those of us who are surviving cancer and other life-threatening illnesses are finding ways to live peacefully in spite of such uncertainty. Above all else, we have turned to faith, strengthening or renewing our relationship with God. We are deeply comforted by the belief that He is at our side every step of the journey. Faith sees us through the darkest hours and longest nights, and has enabled us to transcend pain, crisis, frustration, and fear.

God works through people. Day after day His loving kindness is reflected in the sentiments and actions of friends and family. When we are overwrought they provide stability; when we fear the future they bring us back to the present.

Support groups also help us cope with uncertainty. In those safe harbors we share not only our deepest concerns but also our blessings. We anchor ourselves in mutual love and understanding.

THOUGHT FOR TODAY

Faith brings me blessings even
in the midst of trauma.

> "Nothing is more honorable
> than a grateful heart."
>
> SENECA

You are grateful for the care you've been receiving—that's probably the understatement of the year. Your partner has been at your beck and call constantly. He or she has been tolerant, understanding, and level-headed, during even the most difficult times.

Come to think of it, though, do you sometimes take the relationship for granted? If your partner is occasionally irritable, for example, do you take it personally and become defensive or react insensitively? Perhaps it's time to remind yourself that your partner has a life beyond you, not to mention feelings that can be hurt as easily as your own. Perhaps, too, it's time to reach out and offer *your* help.

Actually, when was the last time you expressed your appreciation? As we all know, a simple "Thanks for all your help!" can do wonders for a flagging spirit.

It's also important to remember that your caregiver is doubtless well aware of your pain and frustration, yet powerless to do very much about it. You can reduce the pressure by trying to limit your complaints and demands. In the final analysis, mutual consideration and respect are qualities of character that can smooth the way ahead for both of you.

THOUGHT FOR TODAY

Gratitude is best expressed
through action.

October 29

"The great art of life is sensation,
to feel that we exist, even in pain."

LORD BYRON

From the very moment we are born, each of us experiences physical pain. Most of the time, fortunately, the pain is relatively minor, transitory, and easily subdued. When we were children our pain could be softened with a kiss. As teenagers and adults we learned to work and play through pain, to casually treat it with an aspirin and perhaps some rest, or to ignore it altogether.

Chronic illness has changed all of that. This is an entirely different kind of pain, deep-voiced yet shrill, one that never disappears entirely but somehow always takes us by surprise.

Where once pain was a casual acquaintance with whom we had only brief encounters, the relationship has evolved. Pain is now a constant companion. We have become intimately familiar with its urgent demands, the sound of its voice, and with what is required to silence it.

Beyond that, strangely and still inexplicably, we sense that we are undergoing beneficial changes because of our relationship with pain. Perhaps our character is being tempered; we have become stronger, more insightful, more understanding, more compassionate.

THOUGHT FOR TODAY

I know you, Pain, and I respect you.
But you will not rule me.

"Pain of mind is worse than pain of body."

PUBLILIUS SYRUS

One of the confounding things about my lupus is that I never know from one day to the next when a flare-up will lay me low. However, there are occasional clues. Sometimes when my immune system is about to go awry, even before the onset of physical symptoms, I feel myself becoming detached from the world around me.

I lose interest in regular activities, such as exercise, reading, or gardening. If I allow the malaise to take hold, before long I don't care if I ever swim another stroke, open another book, or pull another weed. Soon, I hate my work and where I live, and my friends are nuisances.

Needless to say, such states of mind are very disturbing, often more so than the pain and other physical symptoms that follow. They draw me into a swamp of negativity that further compromises my immune system.

Thankfully, it's becoming easier to recognize and accept these thoughts and feelings as actual symptoms of the illness—no less real than a rash, fever, or muscle weakness. Unlike physical symptoms, however, I don't have to treat them, react to them, or act on them. I'm learning to wait for the negative thoughts and feelings to pass. And they do.

THOUGHT FOR TODAY

Is my plummeting mood a barometer of physical changes?

October 31

> "He who knows others is wise.
> He who knows himself is enlightened."
>
> LAO TZU

It has been said that illness is a crucible in which our courage and limits are tested, and where our character traits rise to the surface. Chronically ill people can attest to the aptness of that metaphor.

When we become ill, the traits that first boil upward in the crucible tend to be mostly negative in nature. We brood over past illnesses; we fearfully project into the future; we overflow with anger, self-pity, and self-blame.

This, of course, can be very upsetting, because many of us have considered ourselves to be quite self-aware, with positive attitudes, strong spiritual beliefs, and the ability to handle just about everything. Suddenly it seems that our character liabilities far outweigh our character assets.

However, with the passage of time, the help of others, and a lot of hard work on our part, our positive traits will most certainly rise again to the surface. Moreover, through our illness we will have the opportunity to discover untapped resources of courage and strength. We will be able to put the principles of acceptance and forgiveness into action as never before. We will surely learn much from our illness, and integrate its valuable new lessons into our lives.

THOUGHT FOR TODAY

Illness can put us on an entirely new
path of self-discovery.

November

November 1

> "The will of God will never take you to where
> the grace of God will not protect you."
>
> ANONYMOUS

There are many ways of expressing my faith and trust in God: God is in charge...Thy will be done...God has all power...God is in control. The significance is not in the words I choose, but in the way I bring their reality into my life.

At the start of each day I turn my will over to the care of God. In so doing I affirm my desire and determination to carry the vision of His will into every one of my activities. Wherever I am and whatever I do, my objective is to think and act as God would have me think and act.

I can give my will to God again and again, at any hour of the day or night. Each time I do so it is with confidence and joyous expectation. For I know in my heart that God wants me to heal and thrive; to live joyously, freely, and productively; to love and be loved.

The words I use to express my faith and trust are by no means a reminder to God, but rather a reminder to myself to allow God to work in me, for me, and through me.

THOUGHT FOR TODAY

By seeking and doing God's will,
I live the best possible life.

"It is difficult to say how much men's minds are conciliated by a kind manner and gentle speech."

CICERO

You no longer think of doctors as gods, and you've stopped putting them up on pedestals. That change of attitude has made a world of difference in your relationships with medical professionals. You still respect the fact that doctors have to distance themselves in order to maintain professional objectivity, but you now expect them to be caring and considerate.

What else can you (or should you) expect from a doctor? Your doctor should recognize the fact that what each of you knows is important. While he may have specialized training, knowledge, and experience, your doctor should still be respectful and open to your knowledge, experience, and feelings. For example, when you try to describe what your body seems to be telling you, the doctor should listen carefully— no matter how much trouble you may have putting the symptoms into words.

You should also expect your doctor to be thorough and rigorous, but not mechanical and excessive. Above all, you should expect him or her to be honest and practical, but not indifferent, cold, and hopeless. And it's certainly within reason to expect courtesy, kindness, and even a little empathy.

THOUGHT FOR TODAY

I am an important member of my own healthcare team. Am I being treated as such?

November 3

"I felt it shelter to speak to you."

EMILY DICKINSON

There were ten of us at my first cancer support-group meeting. That night I was the only man. Several minutes after we introduced ourselves, not only the gender difference but various other ones as well became meaningless. The illness we shared created instant closeness, transcending such irrelevancies as age, color, and cultural background. I've been to many such meetings since that time, and it's rare that I ever return home feeling anything less than satisfaction, serenity, and renewed hope.

I can't speak for the others, although I'm quite sure they feel as I do, but I'm convinced that regular participation in such support-group meetings is as important to my overall well-being as any medical consultation or physical therapy program. We can't diagnose symptoms or prescribe drugs, but we are able to alleviate painful feelings of confusion and aloneness. From each other we learn ways to cope with our illness, and to regain control of our lives.

In our support group, we also come to grips with the "why me?" question. It's pretty hard to continue feeling victimized and singled out when you are surrounded by a roomful of caring and empathetic fellow sufferers.

THOUGHT FOR TODAY

Thanks for helping me, and thanks for letting me help you.

"Don't ask the doctor;
ask the patient."

YIDDISH PROVERB

The doctor strides into the examining room just as you are covering yourself with a paper gown that suddenly seems smaller than usual. She listens to your breathing, checks your pulse and blood pressure, and asks how you're doing. You tell her, the best way you can.

Later, on the way home, you clap your hand to your forehead in annoyance. You forgot to mention the most important thing of all, the tingling in your left leg that started last week and has been getting worse. And you also neglected to tell the doctor that the new drug has been causing severe nausea.

Every one of us has been in that same situation. We've caused ourselves needless aggravation and stress by not bringing along the list we drew up or, more likely, by not preparing one in the first place.

Yet such lists (some people call them "personal medical journals") help bridge the communication gap between patient and doctor. They also make it easier to keep track of medications and appointments, to chart the ups and downs of an illness, and overall, to retain a much-needed degree of control over our lives.

THOUGHT FOR TODAY

Guesswork sells me short.

> ## "I am never afraid
> of what I know."
>
> ANNA SEWELL

We don't want to dwell on the illness or make it a full-time preoccupation. It's become clear, however, that keeping a daily medical journal can provide important emotional and physical benefits. No longer do we have to wrack our brain trying to recall the various pieces of the puzzle; trying to fit them into some sort of understandable pattern; trying somehow to make personal decisions from memory; and, finally, trying to communicate it all to a healthcare professional.

Depending on the nature of the illness, we may want to keep a record of changes in our condition, including, for example, sleep patterns, appetite, energy levels, or new symptoms. We may want to describe activities that precipitated a flare-up, as well as times of the day when we felt the worst or the best.

It can also be useful to characterize our pain, regularly making note of its intensity, location, and duration, as well as the steps we took to seek relief. Our daily journal might also include notes on how certain foods affect us, our response to medications, and perhaps most important, a synopsis of each visit and phone contact with our healthcare team.

THOUGHT FOR TODAY
_____

Keeping track keeps me on track.

"Thinking is, or ought to be,
a coolness and a calmness . . ."

HERMAN MELVILLE

A friend used to jokingly ask about my *"obsession du jour."* He knew me so well! I've come a long way since then, but that character flaw sometimes still manifests itself, usually in connection with my health. There's a fine line separating my actual need to deal with a pressing medical problem, and my inclination to become irrationally obsessed with it.

Recently, for example, I noticed a dark spot in the center of my melanoma scar. I had to wait a week to find out if it was just a freckle or a recurrence of cancer. During that week the spot was all I could see, and all I could think about was its life-threatening potential.

As we all know, obsessions can cause great anguish. They distract us from our priorities and frequently harm our relationships as well as our health.

Thankfully, I've learned what to do when my mind obsessively grabs on to a thought and refuses to let go. While I've never been able to "ungrab" an obsession on my own (believe me, I've tried), I've found that God has the power to do so. God alone can remove my obsessions, but only when I am entirely ready to have them removed.

THOUGHT FOR TODAY

Obsessions are injurious to my health.

"We change whether
we like it or not."
RALPH WALDO EMERSON

When we could no longer deny that illness and injury would dramatically change our lives, we were overwhelmed with fear. We were afraid not only of actualities, but also of imagined possibilities: What would become of us? How would we fill our time? Would we lose touch with our friends? How would we find fulfillment? It was as if the rudder had been taken from our lives, and as the result, we would forever after drift aimlessly.

When we gradually became willing to embrace rather than resist the changes that were taking place, our fears diminished greatly. But that was only part of it. The void we had dreaded was soon filled with new discoveries, new learning experiences, new and enriched relationships. We found alternative ways to extract the very best from life.

Along the way, and as an integral part of the process, we gained valuable spiritual beliefs and awarenesses. As an important example, some of us came to believe that whatever takes place in life—not only the obviously good, but also the seemingly bad—is part of a divine plan for our ultimate good.

THOUGHT FOR TODAY

With God's help I will try to erase the
fear and embrace change.

"I want, by understanding myself, to understand others.
I want to be all that I am capable of becoming."
KATHERINE MANSFIELD

You've been aware for several months that something has changed in your relationship with your mother. You can't quite put your finger on it, but she's certainly treating you differently. She doesn't chastise or yell at you, it's nothing like that. It's a much more subtle change, a chilly lacework of innuendoes, pauses, sighs, and long silences.

After wondering at length about your mother's behavior, you now understand what's going on. Your illness has crushed her. Because she's powerless, because she can't love you back to health, she's deeply frustrated. And that painful, fearful frustration comes across as anger at you for getting sick.

It seemed at first that there was nothing you could do to improve the situation. You tried but couldn't make her understand that you didn't bring the illness on yourself. You tried but couldn't alter her behavior or soften her heart.

On reflection, you decide that this is a time when it's far more important for you to be understanding than to be understood, to be loving than to be loved, to be forgiving than to be forgiven.

THOUGHT FOR TODAY

It isn't only about me and my illness. My loved ones are suffering right along with me.

November 9

> "Our greatest foes, and whom
> we must chiefly combat, are within."
>
> MIGUEL DE CERVANTES SAAVEDRA

I've worked for years to raise my self-esteem from rock-bottom levels. Most of the time I'm comfortable with the person I've become, so I know I've made progress.

But when a lupus flare-up forces me to sidestep responsibilities and perhaps spend several days in bed, self-approval sometimes gives way to self-reproach. In fact, my thoughts can become downright self-destructive: "You're being lazy.... You're a burden to your family.... You deserve to feel this way!"

When my self-esteem plummets, it becomes more important to work on my state of mind than to nurse my aching body. I've learned that if I don't shift priorities along these lines, the destructive process could go full circle. In other words, it begins with the physical condition exacerbating the mental condition; it ends up with the mental exacerbating the physical.

I can break out of the circle only by reducing the expectations I've created for myself. My lack of energy may keep me in bed, but that's the best I can do right now. I may need extra help, but that doesn't make me a burden. And, as I move toward acceptance of my physical condition and away from self-deprecation, the healing can resume.

THOUGHT FOR TODAY

When my body attacks me, my mind
doesn't have to go along.

"Is this the poultice for my aching bones?"
WILLIAM SHAKESPEARE

Slowly but surely the drug industry and its distribution network is becoming more efficient and patient-friendly. Most pharmacies now take advantage of computer technology, which enables them not only to track inventory levels accurately and keep up with new product information, but also to record a drug profile for each patient/customer. Such profiles include current and past prescriptions, allergies, physicians' phone numbers, and similar important information.

This is certainly all to the good, but no computer can take the place of a knowledgeable pharmacist who is personally familiar with your health history and the medicines that have been prescribed for you. That's why it's a good idea to develop a close relationship with your pharmacist, and to value him or her as a key member of your healthcare team.

Your pharmacist can alert you and your physician to possible dangerous drug interactions, as well as potential side effects. He or she can also offer personal advice about the relative effectiveness of various over-the-counter drugs, and can help you choose other health necessities. No less important, your pharmacist will recognize you, ask about your health, and take a genuine interest in your progress.

THOUGHT FOR TODAY

There are steps I can take to make my healthcare team more "user-friendly."

> "Speak the language of the company you are in;
> speak it purely, and unlarded with any other."
>
> PHILIP STANHOPE, LORD CHESTERFIELD

During a trip to Germany some years ago, I hurt my back in a fall and had to seek medical treatment. I couldn't speak German, but fortunately I was directed to an orthopedist who understood and spoke a little English.

I was given a fifteen-minute appointment, but it took more than an hour for us to connect, to communicate in a way that made it possible for the doctor to evaluate my injury and provide treatment. With body language, grimaces, pointing, and a great deal of frustration for both of us, I was finally able to let the doctor know how the injury had occurred, what the pain was like, my medical history and current medications, and so on.

The experience made me realize, once again, just how difficult communication with doctors and nurses can be even in familiar surroundings and in established relationships. More important, it demonstrated to me how essential *clear* communication is to proper diagnosis, treatment, and healing; without such communication, very little can be accomplished. Certainly, it helps when the doctor and patient speak the same language, but even then, it's up to us to make sure we are completely understood.

THOUGHT FOR TODAY

Don't give up or give in until your point
is made and understood.

"The holiest of all holidays are those kept by ourselves in silence and apart; The secret anniversaries of the heart."

HENRY WADSWORTH LONGFELLOW

The holidays are fast approaching and we're experiencing familiar stirrings of excitement and expectation. But this year, because we're seriously ill, a part of us wishes that Thanksgiving, Chanukah, or Christmas had already come and gone.

There are some very real problems. We can't travel, and won't be able to participate in traditional family get-togethers. It's obvious that no one in the family feels particularly festive; because of our illness, each day is clouded with uncertainty and it's hard to make holiday plans. Then there are questions which, while speculative, are no less troubling. What kind of celebration, if any, should there be? What if we have to bow out at the last minute? What if we take a turn for the worse?

Let's try to put negativity and speculation aside and remember this: No matter how serious our condition, we are still capable of loving and being loved. Isn't that what celebrations are all about? As for making holiday plans, why not go forward with optimism and faith? If need be, the family's regular celebration can be followed by a special smaller one in our room.

Holidays of course represent different things to different people. But expressions of joy, gratitude, and faith are always beneficial and healing.

THOUGHT FOR TODAY

This holiday season, I will celebrate faith, love, and hope.

> "Freedom is the greatest fruit
> of self-sufficiency."
>
> EPICURUS

I was in the hospital for nine long days following lifesaving surgery. When my brother phoned to find out what time he could pick me up, I burst into tears. It suddenly sunk in that I had lived through the ordeal. I was alive and well, and actually going home!

I expected to feel an even greater sense of relief and gratitude during my first days home. Yet to my surprise I became despondent. My elation gave way to fear, confusion, and an eerie sense of loneliness.

As my spirits continued to plummet, I lashed out at myself for my inappropriate emotions. Was I thankful to be alive, or not? Was I thankful to be home with my family, or not? What was *wrong* with me?

Several days later, a visiting nurse sensed my distress. With some embarrassment, I described my feelings. She smiled understandingly and told me that fear and loneliness were common reactions for patients leaving the hospital. I missed the support of being monitored and cared for by a medical team around the clock, she explained.

The nurse assured me that my uneasiness would soon pass as I became more confident on my own. And, of course, she was absolutely right.

THOUGHT FOR TODAY

Hour by hour, day by day, I am becoming more confident and self-sufficient.

"Being in a good frame of mind helps
one be the picture of health."

ANONYMOUS

There comes a time when those of us with life-threatening illnesses
are ready to hear about our chances. The way this delicate exchange
between doctor and patient is handled can have a profound effect on
our attitude, and influence the type of treatments we choose or reject.
The doctor's manner, as well as the timing and very words he or she
chooses, are almost as important as the prognosis itself.

We as patients have little influence or control over the way a doctor
presents a prognosis. But we do have a great deal of control, and a
clear-cut choice, as to how we respond over time to that information
and use it in our battle for recovery.

There is plenty of research demonstrating the importance of a
patient's attitude and outlook in influencing the course of illness.
If we respond despairingly and pessimistically to a prognosis, and
in effect "give up," we are more likely to become a statistic than
a survivor.

If, on the other hand, we respond positively and courageously; if
we are motivated to fight; if we truly believe that hope is a miracle
medicine, then we have a far better chance of surviving and thriving.

THOUGHT FOR TODAY

To a significant degree, my attitude and
outlook influence "my chances."

> "After the verb 'to love,' 'to help'
> is the most beautiful verb in the world."
> BARONESS BERTHA VON SUTTNER

It's your first day home from the hospital following major surgery. The discharge procedure took four hours and required every bit of your patience and energy. You are exhausted, and it's a relief to finally get into your own bed. But before you can stretch out and have a cup of tea, you receive a succession of phone calls. There are already ten messages on the answering machine and a note on the door.

Relatives, friends, co-workers, they all want to know the same thing. How did the surgery go? How are you doing? What did the doctor say? When can I visit? How can I help? These are caring questions from concerned people, and they deserve to be answered. But it's been an arduous and stressful week and you're at the breaking point.

You can ease the burden by taking up several of those offers of help. Ask one or two friends to return some of your calls and pass along information. Appoint a family member to contact relatives, and a co-worker to spread the word at work.

Finally, select a special friend to help *you* cope emotionally during your recovery. Choose someone understanding and empathetic who can help you get through this difficult and challenging time.

THOUGHT FOR TODAY
_____

Yes, I can use some help.

"People are not disturbed by things,
but by the view they take of them."

EPICTETUS

No matter how optimistic or courageous we are, most of us occasionally become overwhelmed with a sense of hopelessness. We feel alone, adrift, and defeated. Nothing seems to matter anymore.

The actions we have taken in the past to overcome such feelings simply aren't working this time. Neither reading, nor relaxation, nor recreation of any kind changes our state of mind. We have problems connecting with friends and, indeed, feel utterly friendless.

Yet there is always God. Even when we have temporarily forgotten about Him, He remains caring and close-at-hand. Though our connection with God may sometimes be tenuous or even nonexistent, His love for us is constant and unconditional.

God is aware of our pain, but He has not inflicted it upon us. Rather, He has a far-reaching divine plan for our well-being and the well-being of our loved ones.

When we find our way back and reaffirm our faith and trust in God through prayer and meditation, we soon lose our sense of aloneness. We become whole and hopeful again.

THOUGHT FOR TODAY

I will look to God for solace.

November 17

> "Imagination frames events unknown,
> In wild, fantastic shapes of hideous ruin,
> And what it fears, creates."
>
> HANNAH MORE

Like so many chronically ill people, I've been heavily involved with a raft of medical specialists, from dermatologists and oncologists to cardiologists and rheumatologists. And, like so many patients, I have frequently risen or fallen in accordance with my doctor's mood, demeanor, facial expression, or body language.

If his eyes darted nervously, I of course feared the worst. If she sighed deeply and sat down carefully, I knew the biopsy was positive. If he seemed distant and uncommunicative, my palms began to sweat. If he was smiling and upbeat, I was instantly relieved.

Good heavens, the power I gave to a flick of the wrist, a sidelong glance, a clearing of the throat! How foolish of me to read so much into so little!

After putting myself through countless such episodes, it finally dawned on me that healthcare professionals are, first of all, human. They function in a constantly stressful environment; they experience family pressures, living pressures, bad days, and good days.

I've since made it a point, when visiting a doctor, to listen carefully to the words and facts, rather than focus on the manner of delivery. I try to remember that hope, optimism, and faith are *my* responsibility.

THOUGHT FOR TODAY

Concentrate on the message, not the messenger.

"Their cause is hidden,
but our woes are clear."

OVID

There are times when I can pinpoint the exact cause of a lupus flare-up. For example, when I stubbornly overexert myself and spend too many hours gardening in bright sunlight, I can count on a host of severe symptoms. When I go through a lengthy period of extreme emotional stress, it's inevitable that I will be overtaken by fatigue and pain. And when physical exertion is combined with stress (during travel, for instance), it's a virtual certainty that the illness will flare out of control.

I'm frequently on target, but just as often I can make myself crazy trying to figure out the reason for a flare-up. Round and round I go, racking my brain for possible cause-and-effect links: *I haven't been drinking enough water. Could it have been the food? The barometer has dropped; maybe that's a clue. It was hot and humid at the ballgame and I sat too long....*

But enough is enough. I've decided that while it's important for me to remain aware of activities or conditions that can trigger a flare-up, it's equally important to avoid going off the deep end with obsessive analysis and self-blame.

THOUGHT FOR TODAY

Over-analysis can be as damaging
as over-exertion.

> "When we are well it is easy to
> give good advice to the sick."
>
> TERENCE

It is inevitable that some of the people we know will ask probing questions about our illness. So we ought to be prepared to give them concise, factual information. When we do so, it's also a certainty that we will be offered (or perhaps even be barraged with) advice on how to deal with the condition.

Apart from the fact that people often misunderstand certain illnesses, in spite of careful explanations, there is a great deal of folklore about virtually all illnesses. Our friends and loved ones mean well when they urge us, for example, to consult an herbalist, to try off-label prescribing, to radically change our diet, or to stop taking prescribed medications, which, in their opinion, do more harm than good. And it's sometimes tempting to go along with their suggestions in order to gain their approval.

However, no matter how much personal experience a person may have, and no matter how sincere and well-intentioned they may be, we should always think carefully and consult our physician before accepting any advice or altering a treatment plan. If a person puts the pressure on, the best defense is a simple expression of appreciation for their concern.

THOUGHT FOR TODAY

I'm not obligated to follow or even
consider unsolicited advice.

"Troubles are often the tools by which
God fashions us for better things."
HENRY WARD BEECHER

Two o'clock in the morning. The hallway outside of our hospital room is silent, except for the rhythmic swish of a cleaning person's mop. The night has been longer than any we've ever known. If morning does finally come, what new desolation will it bring?

At times like this we feel completely alone, and life seems terribly unfair. How can we be expected to fathom the onset of a life-threatening disease, to accept the painful changes that are still taking place, to go on in the face of such uncertainty? How can we make our way out of this web of despair? Where can we find the understanding, support, and love we so desperately need?

God is ever available and ready to accept the burdens of our hearts. He is close at hand, a breath away, a thought away, a prayer away.

God can help us to accept the inexplicable. He can light the path and lovingly guide us through the shadows of fear and uncertainty.

God will provide everything we need, if only we ask. He will give us courage, strength, and comfort. He will bring us safely through the long, dark night. He will offer bright new hope for tomorrow.

THOUGHT FOR TODAY

I am never alone.

> "When the heart dares to speak,
> it needs no preparation."
>
> GOTTHOLD EPHRAIM LESSING

My friend's elderly mother had fought a long battle against cancer. Several days after her ninety-sixth birthday, she lapsed into a coma. The woman had not prepared a will, nor had she ever revealed her feelings and personal wishes concerning the prolongation of life by artificial means.

For another three months the woman was kept alive with the aid of a respirator and feeding tube. During that time my friend called me almost every day. He was in great emotional distress. Over and over he wondered aloud if he and his two sisters had made the right decision on their mother's behalf.

All I could do was listen and try to empathize; it certainly wasn't my place to offer advice. However, the lesson was clear, and I began taking steps designed to spare my family similar anguish at the end of my life.

Soon thereafter, I talked candidly with my wife, my children, and my brothers. I let them all know exactly what I feel and what I want. I put it all in writing by preparing the appropriate legal documents. Finally, I filed the papers in a safe place, with the expectation that they will gather dust for many years to come.

THOUGHT FOR TODAY

Talk it over, talk it out, make it clear.

"Where there is no choice,
we do well to make no difficulty."

GEORGE MACDONALD

It doesn't happen often anymore, but it does happen. I wake up in the middle of the night obsessed with an unfinished task or unresolved problem. I lie awake for hours. Or I may actually get out of bed—at midnight or 3 a.m., the hour doesn't faze me—and try to repair the washing machine, reread the manuscript, or restore the lost computer file.

For years I've caused myself immeasurable stress because of my unwillingness to live with unresolved issues. The thing is, I know better, of course I do; after all, life is a *series* of unresolved issues. My job is to patiently and peacefully surrender, even though I haven't yet heard from my doctor regarding test results, or from my publisher regarding a book proposal.

If the issues are relatively minor, I try to stop, talk some sense into myself, and adjust my perspective. As for critical and potentially life-altering matters, they are often beyond my control to begin with. Yet even when I can't do anything, there's always one thing I can do: Let go, let God, and trust His will for my life.

THOUGHT FOR TODAY

Acceptance and surrender
equal sanity and serenity.

November 23

"Gratitude is the memory
of the heart"
FRENCH PROVERB

Last night we reminisced about Thanksgiving holidays over the years. For the most part they were warm and pleasant affairs, and we relished the memories. But then we began to think about Thanksgiving this year, and how it will be different in so many ways. For a moment we became choked up and tearful. There was a flash of anger, and this brief but searing thought: What's there to be thankful about?

When the moment passed, the truth came flooding in. Even in the face of illness, pain, family disruption, and cascading change in our lives, there is much to be thankful for. We are thankful for the gift of life and all the wonderful days and years we have had. We are thankful for the dear friends and loved ones who have remained at our side, ever ready with encouragement and support.

We are thankful for the seasons, for laughter and music, for sunrises and sunsets, for the sound of crashing waves.

We are thankful for the spirit of God in our lives, which brings us courage, strength, and purpose. We are thankful for His unconditional love, and for the opportunity to do His will on this very special Thanksgiving.

THOUGHT FOR TODAY

I am blessed.

"What destroys one man
preserves another."

PIERRE CORNEILLE

Chronic illness is often accompanied by severe and intractable pain. Thankfully, pharmacology continues to make progress in this area, providing a wide array of drugs designed to relieve specific types of pain. Yet some people are reluctant to use such medications, despite their suffering, because they are afraid they will become addicted.

From any standpoint, the use of pain medication is an individual and highly personal matter, which is best decided by each of us in accordance with our own background, tolerance for pain, and therapeutic requirements. If you are grappling with this issue, there are some facts worth considering and some questions worth asking.

While some people become addicted by misusing narcotics, tranquilizers, and the like, addiction is usually not a problem when pain medications are used solely and properly for physical needs. That is to say, addiction must include the *psychological* as well as the *physical* component of dependency. Of course, any use of pain medication requires an exit strategy.

If there is any doubt in your mind? Ask yourself: Would I take this medication if I weren't sick and in severe pain? Would I use it to get high? Would I take it to escape from reality?

THOUGHT FOR TODAY

Am I suffering more than necessary?

> "In adversity, remember
> to keep an even mind."
>
> HORACE

If it's true that "belief is biology"—that our thoughts, attitudes, and expectations directly affect our health—then it follows that positive affirmations can enhance the healing process.

An affirmation is an expression of hope, belief, or faith that something we want to achieve, or become, or possess will come to pass. Affirmations can take the form of thoughts, verbalizations, or they can be written.

To create your own healing and empowering affirmations, imagine specific, high-priority hopes or objectives in your life. Then, describe those objectives as if they have already come to pass, or are in the process of being achieved:

I am a whole person. My wholeness transcends my illness, my pain, my body.

There is an abundance of love in my life. I am capable of giving love, and worthy of receiving love.

To make the most of your affirmations, try to keep them in the forefront of your consciousness. Memorize and repeat them often, or write them out and place them where they will catch your eye. Start the day with one or more affirmations, and welcome sleep in the same positive way.

THOUGHT FOR TODAY

I affirm that God's healing grace surrounds me.

"For it is in the giving
that we receive."

ST. FRANCIS OF ASSISI

We've been going to support-group meetings for months, in some cases for years, and we can't say enough about the positive impact our participation has had on our lives. By regularly getting together with others who suffer from the same illness, we have the chance to share feelings we once thought were unique. We get a lot of encouragement, as well as the security and comfort of camaraderie.

Something else happens, too. It happens almost every time, yet it is always unexpected. We find ourselves dwelling less on our own needs and problems (sometimes forgetting them entirely) and devoting most of our attention to the needs and concerns of others.

When someone is distraught about a setback, we jump right in and remind her of all the progress she has made. If a member is in emotional or physical pain, we automatically reach out; we assure our dear friend that the suffering will diminish, as it has for us time after time.

When we leave the meeting, we're grateful that we've been given the opportunity once again to make a difference—in our own lives, certainly, but more importantly, in the lives of others.

THOUGHT FOR TODAY

The getting is in the giving.

November 27

> "There is a great difference between still
> believing something and believing it again.
>
> GEORG CHRISTOPH LICHTENBERG

When the third of my major illnesses was diagnosed unexpectedly and I was scheduled for bypass heart surgery, I began to disclaim everything I had come to believe about a loving God.

Why was God doing this to me? Hadn't I already suffered enough? Was He punishing me for past behavior?

As we all know, such doubts are not uncommon. In the pain and bewilderment of newly diagnosed illness—or for other reasons—we may feel that God has condemned us or betrayed us.

In my own case, these negative feelings faded quickly. The night before surgery, I turned again to God, asking Him for courage and solace. Almost instantly my fears lessened.

The operation was an unqualified success. I reaffirmed then, as I have many times, several reassuring truths about God in my life. He loves me unconditionally. He wants me to be physically, emotionally, and spiritually well, to the greatest extent possible within the unique circumstances of my life.

I've since come to believe that God expects me to learn from my illnesses. In that spirit, I will try to gain strength from them, and to go forward with ever-greater empathy and compassion for my fellows.

THOUGHT FOR TODAY

If God has singled me out, He has done so with
love and in accordance with a divine plan.

"Hard are those questions—
answers harder still."

EDWARD YOUNG

A bedeviling frustration for those of us with chronic illness or pain is a frequent inability to describe accurately what we have, what our symptoms are, and how we feel from day to day. How can we put into words the kaleidoscope of discomfort and disability that can accompany back pain, migraines, multiple sclerosis, or AIDS? How can we help others understand that we may sometimes look healthy and rosy-cheeked even while our bodies ache and our nerves are raw?

At times we get so frustrated that we're tempted to clam up. It seems like too much trouble to explain our condition or even to let on that we're ill. But that's no solution. As we all know, it's vitally important to communicate where we're at and how we're doing.

Whatever your illness or type of pain, it's a good idea to learn in advance how to describe it accurately, clearly, and as simply as possible. That way, when questions are asked, you won't find yourself fumbling for the right words. When it's necessary to explain fluctuating symptoms to your doctor, spouse, co-worker, or friends, here again you can privately rehearse the best way to characterize those symptoms and the degree of their severity.

THOUGHT FOR TODAY

You can reduce frustration and stress by "rehearsing"
the answers before the questions are asked.

> "The mind is like a bow,
> the stronger by being unbent."
> BEN JONSON

"Just relax," the nurse says as she prepares the catheter. "You have to relax," the physical therapist insists as he works to increase the mobility of a painful hip joint. "The test results won't be in until this evening," the receptionist admonishes. "So you might as well relax."

At such times it seems that we are expected to go limp on command, to bring about a state of relaxation by sheer force of will. But of course we can't force ourselves to relax any more than we can force ourselves to fall asleep or blissfully sit through a painful procedure. In fact, when we try to force relaxation we usually become even more tense and agitated.

Since regular relaxation has become a necessity rather than an option in our lives, we're learning how to best achieve this stress-reducing state. No matter where we are or what we are doing, we know that we must first set the stage and prepare ourselves before we can relax. For example, we can visualize a tranquil setting, or a favorite activity. We can focus on our breathing, or a mantra. We can center our thoughts on the presence and power of God.

THOUGHT FOR TODAY

In order to relax, I must first free my mind.

"How impossible it is for strong, healthy people
to understand the way in which bodily malaise
and suffering eats at the root of one's life!"
GEORGE ELIOT

There are a number of things I try to do each day to minimize the physical effects of illness and maximize my emotional stability. I follow a medical treatment program, exercise, pray, and meditate, and keep the lines of communication open. The one thing I do with the *least* regularity is what I probably ought to do most often: work on my self-esteem.

For years prior to the onset of my current illness I had struggled to overcome deep feelings of self-hatred. With the help of many friends and a loving God, I've come a long way. I have also come to understand that building and maintaining healthy self-esteem is a lifelong process.

But chronic illness has a way of eroding one's self-esteem, past progress notwithstanding. In my own case, the physical rigors and emotional distortions of illness are causing me to struggle again with negative self-perceptions, as well as unrealistic comparisons of myself to others. Perhaps most troublesome is the upwelling of old ideas: *I'm a worthless person . . . I deserve to be sick. . . .*

Yes, the challenge has reemerged, but I am committed to overcoming it, one day at a time.

THOUGHT FOR TODAY

I am a sick person becoming well,
not a bad person becoming good.

December

"All my hope for all my help is myself."

MICHEL EYQUEM DE MONTAIGNE

As a young man I believed that people who valued themselves had discovered a remarkable secret that would forever be beyond my reach. It was a mystery to me why my own self-esteem was so low.

It has taken me years to learn that there's much I can do to improve my feelings toward myself. The process is neither a secret nor a mystery but, to the contrary, involves simple and practical actions that are well within my grasp. Here are some of the things I try to do when I become aware that my self-esteem has plummeted:

I focus on my capabilities rather than my disabilities. I give myself credit for what I do well instead of deprecating myself for what I'm unable to do.

I reflect on the progress I've made in specific areas of my life—healing and wellness; relationships with others; spiritual pursuits.

I do the things that make me feel good about myself, from exercise and meditation to helping others.

I counteract negative thoughts by replacing them with positive ones, and by talking out my feelings. Along the same lines, I listen to and *accept* compliments.

THOUGHT FOR TODAY

God values me greatly.
He always has and always will.

> "God grant me the serenity to accept the things
> I cannot change, the courage to change the things
> I can, and the wisdom to know the difference."
>
> REINHOLD NIEBUHR

It's not surprising that the Serenity Prayer is used by millions of people throughout the world. It offers simple and workable spiritual solutions to any kind of living problem.

Many of us use the Serenity Prayer to help us transcend the challenges of chronic pain and illness. When we ask in the first part of the prayer for help in achieving acceptance of the things we can't change, we humbly acknowledge our powerlessness over the calamitous events that have turned our lives upside down. We also acknowledge God's power to help us rise above and beyond those events with grace and serenity.

When we then ask God for the courage to change the things we can, we indicate (as much to ourselves as to God) that we are willing to take responsibility for the actions that are within our capability.

When we ask God in the last part of the prayer to help us determine which things can be changed and which can not, we acknowledge that it's often difficult to make such determinations through intellect alone. We ask God to make His wisdom known to us, to reveal His will for us, to guide us.

THOUGHT FOR TODAY

With God's help, I hope to transcend the challenges of chronic pain and illness.

"Dare to be true: nothing can need a lie:
A fault which needs it most, grows two thereby."

GEORGE HERBERT

It's almost beyond belief, but now both of you are ill. For more than three months your wife has been taking care of you. Now she is so sick that it's necessary for you to try to forget your own suffering and do your best to care for her. You feel so bad for her that you decide, above all, to be on your best behavior, even if that means tiptoeing around reality.

You forbid yourself to do or say anything, anything at all, that might upset your wife. Because you don't want to cause additional stress for her, you avoid expressing frustration or fear about her illness even when such feelings threaten to burst out of you. The problem is, such well-intentioned vows can backfire and put enormous pressure on you—and cause your own illness to worsen.

Certainly you have every right to be upset about your wife's illness. Your lives have been turned upside down once again. Grief, anger, sadness, embarrassment, disappointment—these are normal reactions. It's necessary to face, express, and work through such emotions in order to maintain a healthy relationship and live life as normally as possible.

THOUGHT FOR TODAY

Is my behavior reducing the
pressure or adding to it?

December 4

> "The ideal is in thyself,
> the impediment too is in thyself."
>
> THOMAS CARLYLE

It seems at times that there are two distinct sides of me; I have a spiritual self and an ego-driven self. My egotistical self feels that my case is different, that I'm an exception and deserve special treatment. It insists that everything be done on my terms and at my convenience.

My ego-driven self also believes that it's my responsibility to handle *everything*, including what is clearly beyond my control. It restrains me from asking for help or guidance from others or from God. Not surprisingly, when my ego is in command I am usually quite frustrated and agitated, because I'm not getting my way.

My spiritual self, in contrast, believes that each day of life is a gift, filled with opportunities. It is loving, giving, and capable of feeling deeply connected to others.

My spiritual self is surrendered and accepting. It trusts God, and believes unreservedly that He has a divine plan for my ultimate well-being. When my spiritual self prevails, I am confident, tranquil, and in harmony with my fellows.

THOUGHT FOR TODAY

What self do I choose to be today?

> "Gratitude makes sense of our past, brings peace
> for today, and creates a vision for tomorrow."
>
> ANONYMOUS

We were going along, living life, taking care of business, doing our best, having fun. Everything was pretty much okay. But then one day we experienced an unusual headache, and intense pain that was hard to characterize. In the weeks that followed, new symptoms arose: a rash, overpowering fatigue, loss of appetite. When the tests were concluded and the diagnosis finally made, it seemed certain that nothing would ever be the same again.

Only when serious illness invades our lives do we fully realize the fragility of our personal little worlds. It matters not how carefully we've planned, or how well we've provided for our families. It matters not how hard we've worked, how much we've achieved, or whether we live in cottages of wood or mansions of stone. When the firestorms of illness sweep through, just about everything is leveled and reduced to ash.

But wait; we can still salvage the most precious assets. We have our inner spirit and free will; we have faith and hope; we have the love of our friends, our family, and our Creator. With these assets we can build a new house, live a new life, and transcend any challenge.

THOUGHT FOR TODAY

I will inventory my God-given assets, and
I will be grateful for those treasures.

December 6

"A sudden, bold, and unexpected question doth many times surprise a man and lay him open."

FRANCIS BACON

In a chance meeting with someone we know, the subject of our health comes up. The person wants to know how we are feeling, what it is exactly that we have, and the kind of treatment we are receiving. Some people go so far as to ask about the prognosis for our illness, and may take it even further by offering advice.

Often, we feel cornered and pressured by such encounters. On the one hand, we may be unwilling to respond at all; on the other, we may want to clarify any misunderstanding by answering in clinical detail. As the result of such mixed feelings, we frequently get stuck in uncomfortable and frustrating conversations.

As with so many aspects of illness, planning and preparation can help solve the problem. It's a good idea to decide in advance whom to open up to, and the kind of details we're willing to provide. For example, we may want to give close friends a complete rundown but limit our conversation with a neighbor.

Equally important is learning how to move from the subject of our illness on to something else. A graceful shift is usually as much a relief to the other person as it is to us.

THOUGHT FOR TODAY

Am I learning to say, "So that's the story of my health. Now let's move on to something else"?

"That awful yawn which sleep cannot abate."
GEORGE GORDON, LORD BYRON

At a cancer support-group meeting I noticed a woman fidgeting with a gum wrapper. For more than twenty minutes I watched with fascination as she folded and refolded the tiny piece of paper. During a coffee break, she presented me with the result of her effort: a beautifully crafted miniature origami bird. She told me that she had taken up the art form to overcome the boredom that so often accompanies illness.

The rest of the group took notice and we shared other ways to deal with boredom and feel productive. Here are some of the ideas.

Research a trip to a place you've always wanted to visit, even if traveling seems out of the question for now.

Prepare and regularly update a list of books you want to read and movies you want to see. With a current list at hand, you'll be more likely to follow through.

Consider getting a pet or setting up a small aquarium to help the hours pass more enjoyably when you're not feeling well.

Reach out to someone else. Encourage friends to talk about themselves. Boredom disappears quickly when we get out of ourselves and start thinking about others.

THOUGHT FOR TODAY

Initiative conquers boredom.

December 8

Because of systemic lupus, I require a lot of sleep. The more I get, the less susceptible I am to flare-ups and the better I feel. When I first became aware of this reality, I was delighted; it meant that I still had *some* control over the immune-system disorder and its effects on my life.

But sleep doesn't always come quickly or easily. We all have nights when we toss and turn, when our minds race, or when pain keeps us awake. Then we compound the problem by trying to *force* ourselves to sleep, which creates still more anxiety.

For many months, that's how I reacted, until I realized that my worry over sleeplessness had become a major new source of stress. Now, on nights when sleep doesn't come easily, I don't struggle. I allow myself to be awake, and trust my body to regulate itself.

I find that a good night's sleep often is more the result of what I've done during the day than what happens after I'm in bed. On days when I've been able to exercise, take care of unfinished business, go outdoors—or do whatever is necessary to achieve tranquility—sleep usually comes over me quickly.

THOUGHT FOR TODAY

I can't force myself to sleep,
nor do I need to.

"The wish for healing has ever
been the half of health."

SENECA

We want to get well, desperately so, yet for some strange reason we sometimes balk at a suggested form of treatment. It's not that the new drug or procedure is untested, or one step up from leechcraft; it's just that we have the preconceived notion that it won't work for us. Even when we do go along with a new treatment, we may do so halfheartedly, cynically believing it's really a waste of time and money.

What we forget at such times is that attitude, conviction, and especially faith are catalytic ingredients that can enhance the effectiveness of any drug, procedure, or therapy. The interaction between mind and body is proven and profound; we're already convinced of that. So even if we have reservations about something new, we can only benefit by suspending judgment and simply going forward in faith.

Don't expect miracles, the doctors may tell us. But why not? While there are no guarantees in medicine, and while we may not know with certainty whether a new drug or procedure will prove effective, we know from experience that faith always works.

THOUGHT FOR TODAY

Go forward in faith.

> "As is our confidence,
> so is our capacity."
>
> WILLIAM HAZLITT

Illness has never been my friend, but it has been my teacher. Sometimes I learn new lessons, sometimes I relearn old ones.

Following open-heart surgery some years ago, for example, I completely lost confidence in my cardiovascular system. Irrational fear convinced me that exertion of any kind would flat out kill me. But here's what I soon learned: Belief in my ability to succeed at something greatly influences what I do, how strenuously I do it, and my degree of success. In short, self-confidence is the starting point.

The lesson unfolded when I was a reluctant participant in a cardiac rehabilitation program. During my first session on the exercise bike, fear caused my heart-rate monitor to sound an alarm. Acknowledging my panic, the rehab nurse and other participants assured me that my reaction was normal, and that I was just fine.

With each new session, my confidence grew. Soon I was breezing through twenty-minute workouts without breaking a sweat. I gained confidence in my ability to handle physical exertion. And I was able to let go of the idea that my surgically repaired heart wouldn't hold up. Four months later, I was hiking and whitewater rafting in the rainforests of Costa Rica.

THOUGHT FOR TODAY

First I will believe, then I will achieve.

> ## "I have good hope that there is something after death."
>
> PLATO

We were too busy living to ever think seriously about death and dying. Every few years a friend or relative would pass away and we'd come face to face with loss, grief, and perhaps a certain amount of fear concerning our own mortality. Then time would pass and death would again become remote and too frightening to contemplate.

But death can no longer be ignored. There is still hope, to be sure; we would be lost without it. Yet we are also realists.

The problem is, we know very little about death, and even less about our feelings and beliefs concerning it. Perhaps it's time to sort out those feelings and fears. Perhaps, it's time to come to terms with the mystery of death, to discover what we do or don't believe and what we would like to find out. We can accomplish this by reading and studying, and by exchanging ideas about death and afterlife with friends, loved ones, and spiritual advisors.

While none of us can ever know what happens after we die, the formulation of personal beliefs about death can bring comfort and peace of mind while we are living.

THOUGHT FOR TODAY

Is this a good time to explore my feelings and beliefs about death?

"Simplicity is making the journey of this life
with just baggage enough."
DUDLEY WARNER

You've been up since six and it's not yet noon, and you're already exhausted. You've had to call the insurance company twice to straighten out a bill. The doctor had a hospital emergency, so your nine o'clock appointment became a nine-thirty appointment. That forced you to cancel and reschedule physical therapy.

You still haven't sorted out the day's medications and can't remember whether or not you took the morning pills. Now you have a strange new pain. Is it the illness, or the result of running around all morning?

Sound familiar? There's no question about it, chronic illness has a way of adding all sorts of complications to each and every day. It's hard not to become frustrated and even angry. However, that doesn't mean you have to roll over completely and allow the illness to complicate your *entire* life.

To be sure, the treatment regimen is high priority; you have to follow through. But in the areas where you have a choice—and there are plenty of them—you can strive to keep things uncluttered, uncomplicated, and under control.

THOUGHT FOR TODAY

Wherever and whenever possible,
my goal is simplicity.

"Life is a short affair;
We should try to make it smooth, and free from strife."
EURIPIDES

How can you simplify a life fraught with the unending complications brought on by chronic pain and long-term illness? Where can you begin? Is simplification even possible? It's not only possible, but absolutely necessary, if for no other reason than to reduce stress and maximize your healing powers.

Of course, it's up to you to evaluate your own situation. Let's begin with the telephone, for example. Do you allow phone calls to invade your privacy and rob you of precious relaxation time? If so, decide in advance when and how to limit conversations, when to switch on the answering machine, and when to return calls. The phone should be your servant, not your master.

You can also greatly simplify your life by refusing to take on problems that are not yours. There is no point in getting emotionally involved and squandering energy in situations beyond your control.

Begin to delegate responsibilities at home and at work. You don't have to do everything yourself, and you need not let others pressure you into doing things beyond your capabilities. Finally, learn to "back off" when stress is mounting. Allow yourself the freedom and flexibility to change plans whenever it's necessary to do so.

THOUGHT FOR TODAY

Am I running my life? Or is it running me?

December 14

> "Do not dwell in the past, do not dream of the future,
> concentrate the mind on the present moment."
>
> THE BUDDHA

My focus tends to turn sharply inward when I am experiencing severe pain. The pain demands my complete attention; I not only feel it, but can almost see it within my body. Everything else—my immediate surroundings; people, plans, and prospects; the rest of the world—becomes a blur surrounding one blinding object: *my pain*.

What a narrow and limiting way to live! I don't want to live like that; I refuse to live like that. So what I will try to do is change my field of view. I will direct my senses to the objects, surfaces, and sounds outside of myself, but nearby.

I will study the texture of plaster, the grain of wood, the geometry of window frames. I will focus on fabrics and patterns. I will cock my ear to the hum of a light, the whir of a motor, the tick of a clock. I will lose myself in the shapes and movements of nature.

And after I've done that for a time—a minute, ten minutes, an hour—I will find that the pain has somehow diminished in severity or, no less significantly, that my relationship to it has changed.

THOUGHT FOR TODAY

How do I choose to experience
this minute, this hour, this day?

"If I only have the will to be grateful, I am so."

SENECA

They say we can overcome our malaise by counting our blessings. Gratitude, they suggest, will reduce anger and fear as well as self-pity.

But how can we be grateful when we hurt all the time? How can we be grateful when friends treat us differently and sometimes avoid us entirely? How can we be grateful when we are not able to work or play as we once did? How can we possibly be grateful when we don't know what the future holds for us, or even whether we will survive?

If we are willing to shift our perspective and look with fresh eyes at what the world has to offer, we *can* have feelings of gratitude. We can become grateful for a tender touch, or the smile of a loved one. We can become grateful for nature's glories—a crimson leaf, a golden shaft of sunlight. We can become grateful for each new day.

We can also feel gratitude for our ability to help others, no matter what our physical condition. In that regard, we can discover again that gratitude enriches not only our own life, but the lives of those around us.

THOUGHT FOR TODAY

Yes, there are blessings in my life.

December 16

"There is one spectacle grander than the sea,
that is the sky; there is one spectacle grander
than the sky, that is the interior of the soul."

VICTOR HUGO

The spirit of Christmas is present everywhere. Lights sparkle, music echoes, feelings of joy and peace abound. Our house is decorated, and a fragrant tree has been placed in front of the picture window. It is laden with bright new ornaments and treasured old ones.

This year the family is more tightly knit than ever before, and we have chosen gifts for each other with love and appreciation. One by one they have been set beneath the tree; some are so beautifully wrapped that we can't imagine tearing them open. But of course we will do so eagerly come Christmas morning. After all, the packages are but decorative containers and the gifts are on the inside.

We know that the same is true of our physical bodies and, indeed, of life itself. Yet we sometimes place too much emphasis on outward appearances and fail to recognize and be grateful for the gifts within. We concentrate on physical beauty, or the ruddiness of health, and overlook the inner spirit. We focus on flaws in our neighborhoods, cities, or society as a whole, while the beauty and harmony of God's larger world remains unobserved and unappreciated.

THOUGHT FOR TODAY

Look within, where the real
treasures can be found.

"Begin at once to live, and count each separate
day as a separate life."

SENECA

A friend of mine was diagnosed with a fast-growing cancer a few years ago. He underwent various forms of treatment, to no avail. The oncology team told him there was nothing more they could do, and they promised they would keep him comfortable.

I phoned my friend numerous times over the next year, but was never able to reach him. Then, out of the blue, he called me. He wanted to borrow some guidebooks on Latin America, where I had traveled extensively.

I invited him to my house that afternoon. He was rail-thin and seemed weak, but was otherwise in fine spirits. I hadn't been able to reach him because he had been traveling. He had been to Africa, Russia, and China. Latin America was his next destination. "Some days I'm limited and can't leave the hotel," he told me. "Other days, I have a fabulous time."

When I praised him for his courage, this is what he said: "It has nothing to do with that. I have a choice—to let myself waste away, or to live. Traveling is the thing that has always made me feel most alive. So I'm going to keep doing it as long as I can, a day at a time."

THOUGHT FOR TODAY

I will live today, and each day,
to the fullest.

December 18

"A house is no home unless it contains food and
fire for the mind as well as for the body."
MARGARET FULLER

Now that you are spending more days at home, one way to care for yourself is by enriching your surroundings. How do you feel when you are in the rooms where you spend most of your time? Are they cluttered, noisy, or otherwise uninviting? Or are they warm, welcoming, and comfortable? Do certain areas make you somehow ill at ease? Do others have a relaxing or inspirational effect on you?

If you decide your environment needs changing, you might start by creating what some people call a "serenity corner." This is a special place that can help you feel more secure, relaxed, and spiritually connected. It doesn't matter if the space is a den, bedroom, patio, or a corner of a larger room, so long as it becomes your personal haven for self-renewing activities. This is where you will go to meditate, pray, practice yoga, read, paint, listen to music, or just sit quietly.

The serenity corner can become uniquely yours with very little effort. You can work with lighting, textures, special books, colors, music, aromas, candles, an aquarium, or anything else that helps you feel serene and centered.

THOUGHT FOR TODAY

I will create a special place on the outside,
so that I can more easily create a special
place on the inside.

> "O what a brave thing it is, in every case
> and circumstance of a matter, to be
> thoroughly well informed!"
>
> FRANÇOIS RABELAIS

Tomorrow we're going to be given the test results, plus a rundown on the nature of the disease and a prognosis. There's a part of us that wants to say with bravado, "Give it to me straight, Doc." Another part wants to skip the appointment and pretend it's all a bad dream.

So what *is* the sensible course between these two extremes? What's the ideal balance between knowing too much and not knowing enough?

It's a tough call, but at the very least we want to be given enough information to make intelligent choices about our treatment. On the other hand, if the news is bad we don't want to be hit over the head with it. We don't want a lecture full of statistics and frightening details five minutes after we've been given the diagnosis. Ideally, the doctor will have developed some awareness and sensitivity to the kind of person we, are and how we might react.

Bad news is a terrible, often shocking blow, and patients tend to focus entirely on the negative aspects of their condition. So it's critically important that the bad news be linked, in general terms, to what can be done to help us recover.

THOUGHT FOR TODAY

Ultimately, knowing is less painful
than wondering.

> "I myself must mix with action,
> lest I wither by despair."
>
> ALFRED TENNYSON

When my body tells me to slow down, skip exercise, or get into bed, that's what I usually do. Most of the time, I listen to the admonitions of my illness. But once in a while a special need—emotional, or perhaps spiritual—propels me beyond the boundaries of common sense. Sometimes, in the interest of mental health, I simply have to override my body's messages.

I haven't yet taken an action that has caused real damage, or even a serious setback. I've just stretched my limits, pushing myself to do things my body clearly wasn't up to doing.

Recently, for example, I felt that if I didn't get outside I'd lose my mind. So I spent the afternoon working in my garden. Although my shoulders and elbows ached, I felt like a new man. On another occasion, when I was bone-tired and climbing the walls from pain, I went out to the movies anyway.

What happens when I follow the urgings of my mind and spirit and push beyond physical limits? My attitude improves. I become reconnected to the world. I feel that, at least for one day, I have successfully transcended my illness.

THOUGHT FOR TODAY
Can I do something special today
for my mind and spirit?

> ### "The noblest pleasure
> ### is the joy of understanding."
> LEONARDO DA VINCI

Illness wreaks havoc with relationships, and we all know the reasons. Long-term illness, in particular, causes uncertainty, disruption, disappointment, frustration, stress, resentment, and fear. And that's just part of the picture.

Most of us would give anything to be able to lift these burdens from our loved ones. We would like to remain calm and collected in all situations; to forever avoid sarcasm, criticism, or judgmentalism; to be accepting in the highest spiritual sense; to love unconditionally.

But we are limited by our humanness, and of course can achieve only partial success in accomplishing these goals. What we can do each day, while we gradually move forward on the broader spiritual path, is concentrate on the "little things," which in reality are not little at all.

We can be more affectionate and complimentary. We can listen attentively and empathetically. We can weigh our words carefully in order to avoid insensitivity. We can be more thoughtful, more communicative, more loving.

THOUGHT FOR TODAY

Is it really true that there's nothing
more I can do?

December 22

> "If isolation tempers the strong, it is the
> stumbling-block of the uncertain."
> PAUL CÉZANNE

When we begin to lose self-confidence as the result of illness, it's easy to be funneled downward into a narrowing lifestyle where apprehension regularly overrides enthusiasm. Activities which were once routine in the past can seem formidable; responsibilities we used to handle without a second thought, can seem overwhelming.

The children's birthday party we had planned suddenly seems like far too much trouble. We had promised to prune the fruit trees, but now we fear that we won't be up to it. We're tempted to cancel a weekend trip to visit relatives because we're afraid our presence will dampen everyone's spirits.

If we take just a little time to examine such fearful projections, we'll find that they are almost always exaggerated and groundless. Just because we're under the weather physically, short-term or chronically, that's no reason for our self-confidence to go south as well.

If apprehension rises as we approach a new venture, activity, or responsibility, we can decrease the pressure by reducing the expectations we have of ourselves, by starting out slowly and easily and by doing our very best to remain flexible along the way.

THOUGHT FOR TODAY

Am I shrinking my world needlessly?

"Creativity is not the finding of a thing, but the making of something out of it after it is found."

JAMES RUSSELL LOWELL

A close friend of mine was in a terrible automobile accident several years ago. His broken bones have healed, and he has put his life back together, but he is in constant, intractable pain. He does everything he can to manage the pain and minimize its effects on his life, and his attitude is generally positive. I've learned a lot from him.

One evening over coffee my friend confided, "I've always been a *Reader's Digest*™ kind of guy. I get more out of slogans and one-liners than I do out of long-winded explanations and advice." One of his favorite slogans, he said, is "This too shall pass."

"But it doesn't work very well with this horrible pain," he told me. "The pain is chronic. And I've accepted the fact that it will probably always be part of my life."

He smiled and told me that he had created a new slogan, one more applicable and comforting: *This too is changing, at this very moment.*

"The pain won't pass entirely," he explained, "but it won't always stay the same. Its character changes minute by minute. It's not always intense. And some days are a lot better than others."

THOUGHT FOR TODAY

We can use our creativity to give pain (or anything else) a new face.

> "Perfect good sense shuns all extremity,
> content to couple wisdom with sobriety."
>
> MOLIÈRE

We vowed last week that we would stop talking about our illness, that we would never again say *anything* to *anyone*. Yet for the last fifteen minutes we've been mercilessly spilling our guts to a neighbor who casually asked, "How's it going?"

We promised ourselves that we would rigorously follow our diet and exercise plan. The first week we went overboard, eating little and doing far more than we were supposed to. The second week we swung all the way back to our old habits of too much high-fat food and no exercise at all. The scenario has been much the same for pain management: We've gone from the one extreme of obsessing about our pain to the other of trying to ignore our pain entirely.

Such an all-or-nothing approach to illness-related issues can cause a repeated sense of personal failure. It can also be detrimental to progress overall. Thankfully, however, we are becoming ever more aware of our tendency to operate at extremes, and this awareness will surely move us closer to the goal of balance in all areas of life.

THOUGHT FOR TODAY

If my goal is "*perfect* balance," then I'm still thinking in extremes.

"Have you seen God's Christmas tree in the sky,
With its trillions of tapers blazing high?"

ANGELA MORGAN

This year Christmas comes at a special time in my life. Personal difficulties and challenges abound, yet everything in my world shines with a wondrous light. In order to make the most of this day, I will take a few moments to ponder the true meaning of Christmas, and to prepare myself for the day emotionally and spiritually.

I will put aside all expectations, so that I may fully experience the day as it unfolds. I will not dwell on what Christmas once was, or what it should be. Rather, I will accept and appreciate it exactly as it is.

I will honor my personal needs while doing my best to avoid self-centeredness, particularly self-pity. I will focus on what I can do for others instead of on what I feel should be done for me. I will reach out to my friends and loved ones in whatever ways I can. I will be motivated by feelings of love, kindness, warmth, and understanding.

My circumstances may not be as I would have wished, but that need not prevent me from celebrating peace, joy, and harmony. Through my thoughts and actions, I will try to show my gratitude for God's glory and grace.

THOUGHT FOR TODAY

I will celebrate giving, and goodness,
and the glory of God.

December 26

"We arrive at the various stages of life quite as novices."

DUC DE LA ROCHEFOUCAULD

Your husband has prepared some of your favorite foods, but you're not eating today. You won't let him bathe you or change the sheets. You feel edgy and somewhat combative. You're not sure what's going on. And you wonder, "Is it me, is it the disease, or is it the medication?"

Those of us with chronic and debilitating illnesses know how confusing and frightening such dilemmas can be. It's sometimes a major challenge to tell the difference between our emotional responses to a disease and our actual symptoms from the illness or various drugs.

This is especially true when dealing with illnesses such as AIDS that can affect the central nervous system and cause personality changes. Are we upset and depressed because we're "sick and tired of being sick and tired"? Or is our depression a new manifestation of the disease process?

There are no simple answers. Clearly, we need to learn as much as we can about the physiological and psychological symptoms of the illness, as well as the side effects of the drugs we're taking. That knowledge will help us understand our reactions and behavior. No less important, we should try not to overreact or panic when new symptoms or feelings surface. Now more than ever, we need to be compassionate and patient with ourselves.

THOUGHT FOR TODAY

Give yourself a break.

> ## "Every change of scene becomes a delight."
> SENECA

When you are bedridden for days or weeks and too sick to do anything requiring physical or even mental exertion, it's hard to know how to fill the time. It would be nice to catch up on your reading, but when you are feverish or in pain it can be difficult to focus, let alone absorb and comprehend.

The first few times that I was bedridden, I ended up doing what most of us do: TV "channel surfing," aimlessly and endlessly. I became hooked on game shows, then talk shows, and finally sitcom reruns. Before long I didn't even have to check the TV listings to know what was on.

Soon my daily routine became dehumanizing, degrading, and depressing. It was necessary to make some changes.

First, I decided how many hours of television I would allow myself to watch, and I vowed to choose programs that were substantive and enriching, or at least out of the ordinary. Next, I had friends provide me with lists of their favorite movies, instructional videos, and audio books. I borrowed, rented, or purchased the ones that seemed most interesting, and was soon able to get off my treadmill of mindless monotony.

THOUGHT FOR TODAY

What I choose to do with my time is just as important now as it ever was.

"It is now high time
to take heart of grace."

THOMAS BECON

Long before I became chronically ill, I learned that one can live well and productively even when burdened with pain and disability. The lesson came from a colleague and dear friend who, in his thirties, developed lung cancer.

During the first several months of treatment he reacted as many of us do. The illness was central to virtually every thought and action and, in fact, seemed to become his identity.

But then, for no apparent outward reason, he underwent a profound change in attitude and outlook. When we were together, his conversation almost always focused on spirituality, nature, his personal interests, and pleasant memories of past experiences. As sick as he became, my friend refused to see himself as a victim. He maintained his dignity, enjoyed the simple things, and continued to reach out with emotional support to friends in need.

He is gone now, and I think of him often. I may never be able to manage my illnesses and minimize their effects on my life as gracefully as he did, but I do my best to follow his example.

THOUGHT FOR TODAY

I can live well again.

> "So great was the extremity of his pain and anguish,
> that he did not only sigh but roar."
>
> MATTHEW HENRY

Pain doesn't simply "hurt," but has many dimensions. Pain wears us down emotionally and exhausts us physically; it also confuses us, causing erratic thinking and behavior.

We do our best all day long to tolerate the pain and carry on in spite of it, but as evening approaches our nerves have become frayed and we are bone-tired. All too often, at that point, we explode at the people we care about the most. Then we feel guilty, which adds to the stress.

The evening letdown and subsequent outburst can become a regular occurrence, taking a heavy toll on the entire family. However, once we recognize the pattern, as well as its causes and consequences, we can do something constructive about it.

First, we can discuss the situation with family members, explaining how chronic pain, tolerated all day, causes fatigue and irritability. We don't expect to be handled with kid gloves, but we do need understanding and patience.

For our part, we resolve to do what we can to break the cycle. We try to avoid problem-solving and serious discussions at day's end, for example. And we take actions (a short walk, a nap, meditation) which help us release pressure and regain inner peace.

THOUGHT FOR TODAY

I can defuse pain-generated explosions.

> "If you think about disaster, you will get it.
> Brood about death and you hasten your demise.
> Think positively and masterfully, with confidence and
> faith, and life becomes more secure, more fraught
> with action, richer in achievement and experience."
>
> SWAMI VIVEKANANDA

We've all known people who angrily disavowed their spiritual beliefs when they experienced major adversity. We heard their arguments and even understood their feelings.

"My parents were right after all. God *is* harsh and punishing." "I used to think He cared about every single one of us. But now I'm probably going to die. Does He know that? Does He care?"

Some of us had these same thoughts when illness overshadowed our lives suddenly and unexpectedly. The irony, of course, was that we were ready to alienate ourselves from God at precisely the time when we needed Him most.

After the initial shock passed and we saw that acceptance was our only choice, we were able to rebuild our faith. We came to believe again, at a deeper level, that God is a constant wellspring of guidance and strength, always there for us when we are uncertain and fearful. We saw, more clearly than ever, that He can bring calm and order into our lives when everything around us is in disarray, and when we ourselves are in emotional turmoil.

THOUGHT FOR TODAY

My faith may sometimes waver, but
God's love for me is constant.

"Ring out the old, ring in the new,
Ring, happy bells, across the snow;

The year is going, let him go;
Ring out the false, ring in the True."

ALFRED TENNYSON

Like many people, I usually do some serious reflecting at year-end. This year I found myself dwelling negatively on unpleasant events and emotions I had experienced during the last twelve months. I began to feel sorry for myself, then I became angry and depressed. Before long I was dreading the year to come.

My initial mental review focused on things like medical bills, opportunities I had missed because of illness, my self-image problem, and the pain I had suffered. In short, my review was not only self-pitying but also self-centered.

So I'm going to start again. This time I'm going to think about other people, especially the ones who stand by me no matter what. I'll focus on the year's blessings: sunny and pain-free days, restful nights, successful vacation travel. I'll reflect on the books I've read and enjoyed, the movies I've seen and loved, the new friends I've made.

I'll try to remember all the things I've learned this year; the challenges I've overcome; the help I've received; the healing that has taken place; and the love that has flowed.

THOUGHT FOR TODAY

I resolve to be grateful for this day, for the life I have lived, for the life yet to be.

Index

About the Author

No stranger to chronic illness and pain, the author has survived malignant melanoma and coronary artery bypass surgery, and is challenged by lupus and osteoarthritis. He has been in recovery since 1970 and chooses to remain anonymous in accordance with twelve-step recovery program principles. J. S. Dorian is a pseudonym.

The author has written several successful books with a combined total of more than one and a half million copies in print, including *A Day at a Time*, a classic work in recovery literature, *A New Day*, *A Time to Be Free*, *At My Best*, and *Tranquility*. His books have been translated in countries throughout the world.